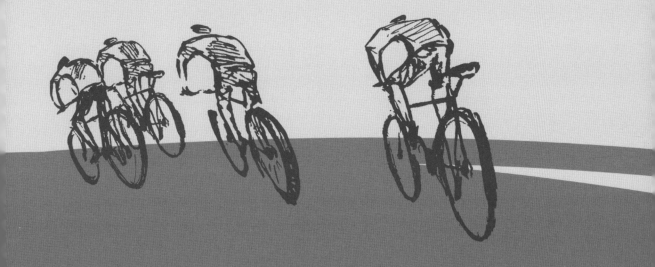

the
cyclingchef

BLOOMSBURY SPORT
Bloomsbury Publishing Plc
50 Bedford Square, London, WC1B 3DP, UK

BLOOMSBURY, BLOOMSBURY SPORT and the Diana logo are trademarks of Bloomsbury Publishing Plc

First published in Great Britain 2021

Food photography by Clare Winfield
Food styling by Megan Davies
Other photography by Daniel Gould
Design by Sian Rance for D.R. ink
Images on pp. 8–9, 18, 24–5, 44, 68, 96, 102–3, 118, 124–5, 144, 176–7, 178 and 186–7 © Getty Images

The information contained in this book is provided by way of general guidance in relation to the specific subject matters addressed herein, but it is not a substitute for specialist dietary advice. It should not be relied on for medical, health-care, pharmaceutical or other professional advice on specific dietary or health needs. This book is sold with the understanding that the author and publisher are not engaged in rendering medical, health or any other kind of personal or professional services. The reader should consult a competent medical or health professional before adopting any of the suggestions in this book or drawing inferences from it. The author and publisher specifically disclaim, as far as the law allows, any responsibility from any liability, loss or risk (personal or otherwise) which is incurred as a consequence, directly or indirectly, of the use and applications of any of the contents of this book. If you are on medication of any description, please consult your doctor or health professional before embarking on any fast or diet.

Bloomsbury Publishing Plc does not have any control over, or responsibility for, any third-party websites referred to or in this book. All internet addresses given in this book were correct at the time of going to press. The author and publisher regret any inconvenience caused if addresses have changed or sites have ceased to exist, but can accept no responsibility for any such changes

A catalogue record for this book is available from the British Library
Library of Congress Cataloguing-in-Publication data has been applied for

ISBN: HB: 978-1-4729-7864-6; ePUB: 978-1-4729-7855-4; ePDF: 978-1-4729-7856-1

2 4 6 8 10 9 7 5 3 1

Typeset in ITC Century by D.R. ink
Printed and bound in China by C&C Offset Printing Co., Ltd.

Bloomsbury Publishing Plc makes every effort to ensure that the papers used in the manufacture of our books are natural, recyclable products made from wood grown in well-managed forests. Our manufacturing processes conform to the environmental regulations of the country of origin.

To find out more about our authors and books visit www.bloomsbury.com and sign up for our newsletters

ALAN MURCHISON

the cyclingchef

Recipes for Getting Lean and Fuelling the Machine

BLOOMSBURY SPORT

LONDON · OXFORD · NEW YORK · NEW DELHI · SYDNEY

Contents

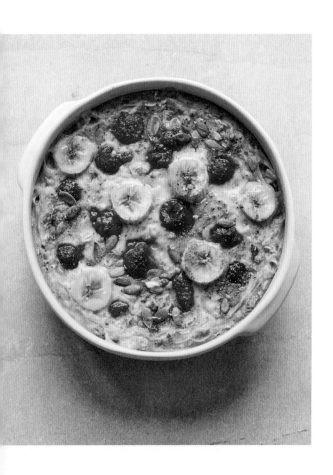

Hard days: Fuelling the machine   150

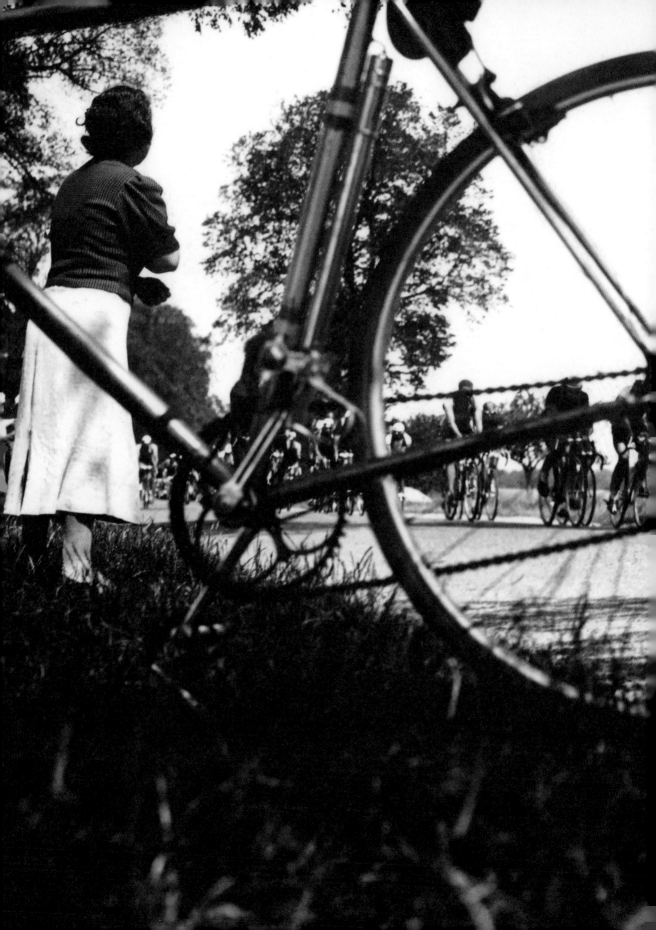

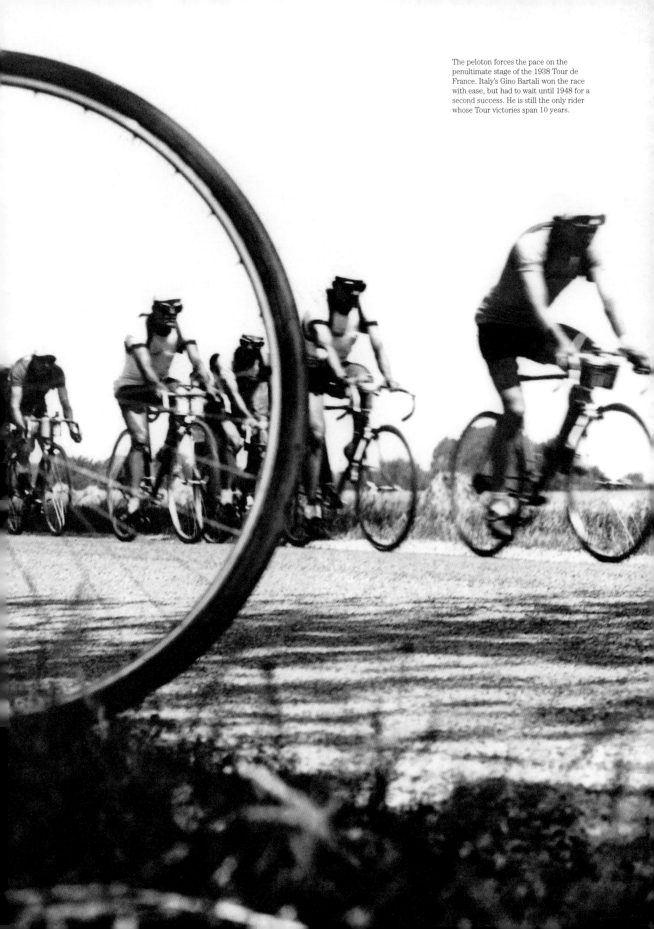

The peloton forces the pace on the penultimate stage of the 1938 Tour de France. Italy's Gino Bartali won the race with ease, but had to wait until 1948 for a second success. He is still the only rider whose Tour victories span 10 years.

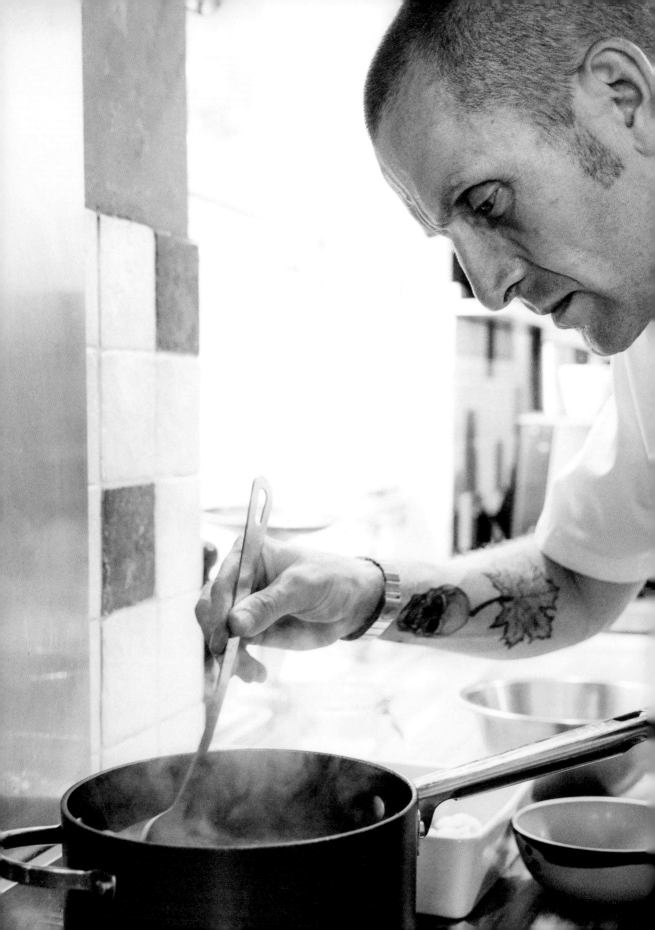

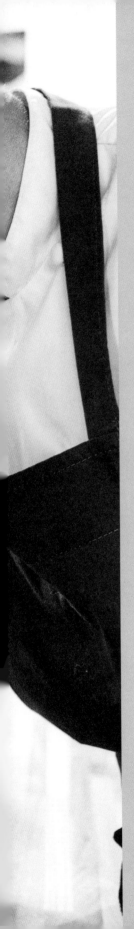

Introduction

What I love about cycling is probably exactly what you love about cycling. It's going full gas and burying myself. It's testing my physical capabilities, smashing my PB and getting the better of my mates. None of that comes easy, but what you need to do to achieve it is actually pretty simple. To maximise your cycling potential, eat well, train well and sleep well. Eating the right stuff is key because it ensures your body has the right levels of all nutrients, not just for those big race days, but for ordinary week-in, week-out training sessions, too. Without correct nutrition, your body won't be able to make the most of those training sessions and when it comes to competitions, the energy reserves just won't be there.

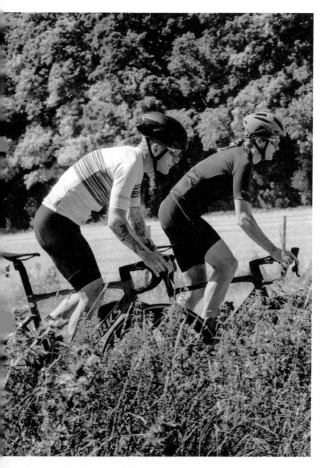

Balancing food consumption with training load is key for cyclists attempting to improve performance. Planning your diet is not just about race days, it also helps ensure that training rides are as effective as possible.

However, as well as eating for pleasure – and I will always advocate that – you need to eat optimally. As a cyclist, you can consume fantastic quality food and have the most amazing diet, but if that isn't balanced with the right training load, you can still end up piling on the pounds, which will slow you down on the bike. I know from personal experience that weight management is one of the most complicated areas of performance for cyclists to address and the recipes in this book have been created with that very much in mind. They're divided into six sections, each corresponding to a phase of the training year and the different types of activity you'll be undertaking, but I've still kept flavour at the forefront.

Off-season

In my view, during the off-season you can afford to take the brakes off a bit and enjoy dishes like my Boozy beef casserole (*see* p. 38) or, for afters, my Coconut, lemon curd and gingerbread chia puddings (*see* p. 42), because, to be honest, the food choices you make in December are unlikely to affect your key performances in June. As they say, a little of what you fancy does you good and a swing of a few kilos won't harm you. In fact, if you've been racing at the low end of your weight range, it will probably be beneficial to 'top back up' over the winter months. A little free-wheeling now also makes it easier to renew your focus on what you eat and your self-discipline later on.

Pre-season

When pre-season training starts, it's time to get more serious about what you consume, but once you've finished up all the Christmas chocolate, don't go cold turkey! Take back control gradually by incorporating some structure into your diet and re-establish good food habits – basically, that means cutting down on snacking. Make yourself more aware of what you're eating by keeping a food diary (the MyFitnessPal app (www.myfitnesspal.com) is helpful for tracking your food intake). If that doesn't work, dig out last summer's kit and put it on. That should shock your system into backing away from the biscuit tin fast! The recipes in this section contain lower levels of carbohydrate to help you focus on your body composition – your proportion of muscle to fat – and get back on track. The Spicy roast parsnip soup (see p. 56) is particularly delicious, or why not give my Baked cod with tomato ketchup – yes, that's ketchup – and tarragon relish (see p. 59) a go?

Soft-pedalling days

Food-wise, soft-pedalling days can be quite tricky as your energy levels – and hence what you need and want to eat – can vary hugely, depending on factors such as the previous day's training, how much sleep you've been getting and external stresses (yes, we all have them). On these days you might experience some hunger pangs, but as you won't be expending the calories, take care to avoid the temptation to overeat. In principle, you need to knock back the carbs and ramp up the protein, but Baked ginger and sesame sea bream 'en papillote' (see p. 88) or Sweet potato tortilla, Vittoria-style (see p. 82) will help you do just that, or try my Roasted butternut squash and beetroot salad (see p. 77). I'd also advise you to pile your plate high with greens and leafy salad to fill yourself up. A cup of coffee or two can also be great for suppressing the appetite, too. Just make sure you don't overdo the coffee. I have to admit,

If your diet isn't balanced with the right training load, you can still end up piling on the pounds, which will slow you down on the bike.

When you hit the hard days, it's really important to face them 'fully loaded' – assuming you don't want to have to call a taxi to get you home, that is!

like many cyclists, I'm a bit of a coffee monster. However, some people can get the shakes and feel dehydrated, depending on tolerance levels.

A brief word about quantities: if you consistently consume too much – an additional spoonful of oats at breakfast, one more slice of bread at lunch or too much rice with your main mean – you'll won't shift the kilos in the first place or, having worked so hard to reach your goal weight, you'll quickly start to put the pounds back on, so weigh out what you eat and be strict with yourself when it comes to portion control.

Pre-race

Once the season is underway, the 24 hours prior to racing or any other key event are hugely important. The way to go is high-energy, high-carb, low-fibre meals that are easy to digest in the run-up to the race start. Sweet and spicy chilli salmon (*see* p. 107) is a good one here, or my quick and easy take on spaghetti carbonara, Pasta 'Barlow' (*see* p. 113) or Old-school chicken, apricot and pomegranate pilaf (*see* p. 114). You can undo all your previous good work by taking your eye off the ball – or the wheel in front – so practise preparing your pre-race food just as you practise every other part of your preparation.

Medium days

What do I mean by medium days? You know, those days when you're happy to roll along in the middle of the pack. The days when you're serious about clocking up the miles and your training schedule says you need to push yourself at some point, but not too much and definitely not to the edge of exhaustion. These recipes are all like that – pretty easy-going and well-balanced. There are some great breakfast ideas here, including Cherry coconut granola bars (*see* p. 130), a nice take on Teriyaki chicken (*see* p. 138) and the Glazed gnocchi, roasted red pepper, tomato and smoked chorizo (*see* p. 136) is highly recommended, but then all these recipes are highly recommended or they wouldn't be in the book!

Hard days

When you hit the hard days, it's really important to face them 'fully loaded' – assuming you don't want to have to call a taxi to get you home, that is! Put further weight loss out of your mind and don't under-fuel. There's no point in being a few kilos lighter if you can't finish the session. Hard days are critical to pushing up your power, but ultimately, you can only train as hard as you can recover and your diet is integral to that recovery process. Full gas sessions will use up to 1 gram of carbohydrate per kilo of bodyweight per hour, so embrace the carbs. My Cherry 'baked well' oats (*see* p. 154) will set you up right, while Pineapple and ginger sweet and sour (*see* p. 162) is just what you need after a day in the saddle.

I may be a Michelin-starred chef, but I'm also a serious cyclist and I understand that cooking from scratch, if possible with fresh ingredients, may be the last thing you want to do when you unclip and dismount, so plan your food intake with the same precision as you plan your training schedule. I've worked with bike-riders at all levels, amateur and pro, and believe me, that extra effort will pay off. This book gives you a roadmap for significant sustainable weight reduction and I hope the recipes, which are practical and uncomplicated, will inspire you to get lean and boost your performance on the bike.

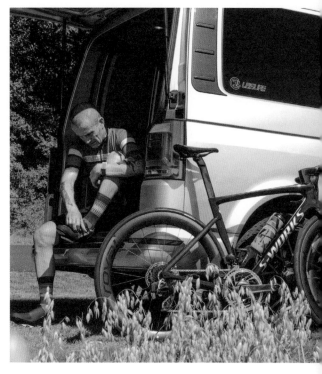

Preparing for a race is a serious and meticulous business. Remember to pay as much attention to your pre-race consumption as you do to your clothing and bike.

Power to Weight Chart

The power to weight chart, right, illustrates the impact of changes to body weight on cycling performance. I used this chart to undertake a highly unscientific experiment on myself and the results were startling – and a large part of the inspiration behind this book.

I performed three standard power tests – 1-minute, 5-minute and 60-minute efforts – and plotted myself (at my then current weight) on the table. This is a well-known chart for classifying cyclists. I then looked at what would happen if I lost or gained a few kilograms. In the 60-minute test (or functional threshold power test (FTP) – *see* p. 22) at 82 kg my power numbers classed me as 'very good', at 74 kg I was 'excellent' and as a lightweight 70 kg I would be classed as 'exceptional'. However, there is one very important caveat. This looks like a win-win situation, right? Drop weight then get faster? Not always.

The assumption made by this chart is that weight has been lost or gained without any impact on power output, but this is not always the case. If weight loss comes at the cost of your power, then you could actually end up being hungry, miserable and slower – and possibly quite unwell. It is all about finding that sweet spot: a sustainable weight where you feel energised, fit and strong. For me that is the middle weight of 74 kg; at 82 kg I felt sluggish and heavy and at 70 kg I felt weak. At my ideal 74 kg I am able to sustain my training load and also feel energised in myself. The recipes in this book will help you discover your optimal weight.

Pretty shit hot

National level

Fastest rider in your region

Fastest rider in your county

Fastest rider in your town

Fastest rider in your street

Fastest rider in your household

All the potential

Men			Women		
1 min	**5 min**	**60 min/FTP**	**1 min**	**5 min**	**60 min/FTP**
11.5	7.6	6.4	9.3	6.6	5.7
11.25	7.4	6.2	9.1	6.4	5.5
11	7.2	6	8.9	6.2	5.3
10.8	7	5.8	8.7	6	5.2
10.7	6.9	5.7	8.6	5.9	5.1
10.5	6.7	5.6	8.5	5.8	4.9
10.2	6.5	5.4	8.3	5.6	4.8
10	6.2	5.2	8.1	5.4	4.6
9.8	6	5	7.9	5.2	4.5
9.5	5.8	4.9	7.7	5	4.3
9.3	5.6	4.7	7.5	4.9	4.1
9	5.4	4.5	7.4	4.7	4
8.8	5.2	4.3	7.2	4.5	3.9
8.6	5	4.2	7	4.3	3.6
8.4	4.8	4	6.8	4.1	3.5
8.2	4.6	3.8	6.7	3.9	3.4
8	4.4	3.6	6.5	3.8	3.2
7.7	4.2	3.5	6.3	3.6	3
7.5	4	3.3	6.1	3.4	2.8
7.2	3.8	3.1	5.9	3.2	2.7
7	3.6	2.9	5.7	3	2.5
6.8	3.3	2.7	5.5	2.8	2.4
6.6	3.1	2.6	5.3	2.6	2.2
6.3	2.9	2.4	5.1	2.4	2
6.1	2.7	2.2	4.9	2.2	1.8
5.9	2.5	2	4.7	2	1.6
5.6	2.3	1.8	4.6	1.9	1.5

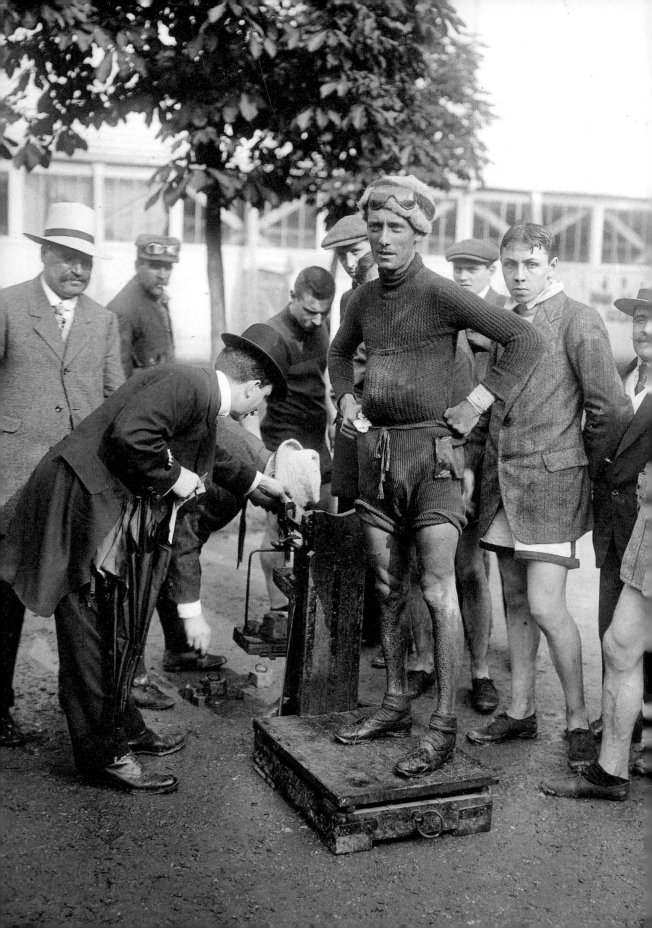

What's to Lose?

How do you know when you need to lose weight? Is it when you can feel your belly gently resting on the top tube as you reach for the drops? Or when last year's jersey begins to feel more and more like a skinsuit? Or maybe you find yourself in a good position in the club run, right up until you hit that climb and start to struggle to cling to the back of the bunch? Whichever scenario it is, you're probably right. It's time to shed a kilo or two – and you're not going to do that by buying a new lightweight stem.

A rider has his weight checked after finishing the 1912 Tour de France. Weighing yourself before and after a ride can help you keep track of your hydration levels.

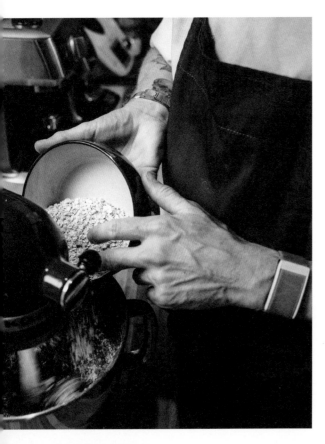

Food choices are vital to performance. Cooking from scratch with fresh ingredients allows you to enjoy your food as well as giving you control over what and how much you consume.

What's the optimum weight for a serious cyclist? It's an impossible question to answer. A Grand Tour winner could be 60 kg, at peak fitness and able to sustain his form for three gruelling weeks on the road, while an Olympic team pursuit rider could be 85 kg, also at peak fitness and able to achieve sub 3 minutes 50 on the track once every four years. Both are endurance riders and both are at the top of their game.

Successful cyclists really do come in all shapes and sizes, but they're generally very lean, with climbers and all-rounders tending to be smaller and lighter than sprinters and time triallists. At 1.90 m tall, Sir Bradley Wiggins is the tallest winner of the Tour de France and in 2012, when he won the Tour, he weighed 69 kg. At 1.86 m, Chris Froome is slightly smaller than Sir Brad and his racing weight of 66 kg is also slightly less, but sprinter and regular winner of the green jersey, Peter Sagan, is only a couple of centimetres shorter than Froome, yet weighs considerably more – 78 kg! There is perhaps slightly less variation in what women cyclists weigh – Marianne Vos and Annemiek van Vleuten are both 1.68 m tall, the former is 58 kg, the latter 62 kg – but both are undoubtedly lean.

Performance factors

It's true that there are a number of factors that determine your cycling performance. Muscle strength, aerobic endurance (how efficiently your body supplies nutrients and oxygen to the muscles), and timely nourishment and hydration are among them, but body weight not only affects many of these, it is a key factor in itself. However, as detailed by many psychologists and nutrition experts, body weight is a complex issue. You might think you look overweight when you're not, or you may be blaming bad performances on excess grams when the cause lies elsewhere, so ask yourself if you really need to lose any weight at all.

A commonly used measure to define a healthy weight is your BMI (body mass index). This is found by dividing your weight by your height squared, so if you weigh 65 kg and are 1.75 m tall, then your BMI is 65 ÷ (1.75 x 1.75) = 21.22. The accepted range for 'normal' is 18.5 to 25,[1] although that's not particularly useful for athletes, because high muscle mass means they weigh more, which skews the calculation and can lead them to exceed the upper end of the range.

Of far more use to us is to look at lean body mass: how much of your weight is muscle and how much is fat? A certain amount of fat – 3 per cent for men, 12 per cent for women – is essential for health, but excess body fat increases the amount of work required to move the body without adding to the body's ability to generate energy. A healthy body fat percentage is 15–17 per cent for men and 18–23 per cent for women, but professional athletes have percentages even lower than these.[2]

There are various methods of measuring body fat. The most accurate results can be achieved by the hydrostatic underwater weighing tests, body pods or DEXA scans available at a cost from some universities or specialist facilities. If you are interested in getting tested professionally, bodyscanuk.com offers DEXA scanning to monitor body composition, whereas one of the leading sports science centres in the UK, Loughborough University, offers body composition assessments using the skin fold caliper method.[3] However, for our requirements, a body composition monitor will suffice. Your body fat percentage should give you a guide to how much weight loss you should aim for. This ultimately depends on your ambitions as

Successful cyclists really do come in all shapes and sizes, but they're generally very lean...

a cyclist. If you are happy to give a good account of yourself on a club run on a Sunday then you might be happy to aim for 15 per cent (perhaps 20 per cent for women), whereas a competition rider might aim to go a few percentage points lower. If you weigh in around 70 kg and need to lose 5 per cent body fat, that amounts to a loss of 3.5 kg. However, you could lose up to a kilo in water before any fat disappears and, if you're not careful, you might lose muscle mass instead and that's a real no-no, so look to your monitor as much or even more than your scales.

Power output

Now, it's time to get on a bike: a stationary bike with a power meter (many of the smart turbo trainers have a power meter built in). Warm up for a few minutes and then measure your average power output. Be aware that the reading can change depending on whether you're timing a 10- or 20- or 60-minute ride, which in turn depends on your stamina. This will give you a pure power reading and pure power indicates how fast you could ride on a flat road. You may be giving your rival a 10 kg advantage, but for that 10, 20 or 60 minutes, if you have more power on the same bike in the same conditions, you will be the faster rider.

The other performance-related test you'll want to look at with your coach is a functional threshold power (FTP) test. For this, you'll need a power meter, heart rate monitor and cycling computer. FTP is the average power that you can produce over 60 minutes. It's measured in watts,

expressed as watts per kilo (the power you produce divided by your weight) and is based on the theory that the lighter you are, the less power you need to ride at the same speed. If you're focused on training for a particular event, you can track your progress by measuring your FTP once a month – if the number rises and your weight remains static or, ideally, decreases, your fitness will have improved.

Here comes the but… There are two major forces riders have to contend with and the first is resistance, particularly wind resistance. Serious cyclists analyse their CdA or 'drag area'. It's more maths, and we don't need to go into the details here, but how you position yourself on the bike and what equipment you use can make a real difference. Understanding CdA is a constantly evolving area of performance. However, if you can knock out 6 watts per kilo for 20 minutes but ride your bike full meerkat, then you're going to be slower than a rider who puts out 5 watts per kilo but has a world-class CdA (that's why, as they say, power is vanity, aero is sanity). It's common sense that the less bulk you present to the wind – or the more aerodynamic you are – the less resistance you will experience and, although it's not necessarily a linear one, there's clearly a relationship between bulk and weight. In basic terms, this means the leaner you are, the less wind resistance you're going to encounter.

As soon as you hit an incline, you face another factor: gravity. Your weight is now an issue and can cost you minutes on a serious climb. For this reason, we need another measurement, called power to weight ratio (PWR) – the real golden number of cycling. PWR is calculated by dividing your average power output by your weight: the higher the number, the stronger the rider. For example, imagine you measure your power output at 280 watts and your rival hits 250 watts. You weigh 80 kg and therefore have a PWR of 3.5 watts per kilo, while your rival only weighs 70 kg, so has a PWR of 3.57 watts per kilo. Your rival, therefore, has the upper hand, and the longer and steeper the climb, the bigger the advantage they will have. You may gain a small benefit on the descent, but that only lasts a fraction of the time of the climb.

To put yourself on even terms, you have three alternatives: increase your power output with no change to your weight; decrease your weight and maintain your power output; or go for the double whammy – increase your power and decrease your weight. For many riders, losing weight is the easiest option and it really can make a difference. It depends on the length of the climb, but on a 10 per cent gradient, a loss of 10 kg can result in a 10 per cent gain in time. Food for thought…

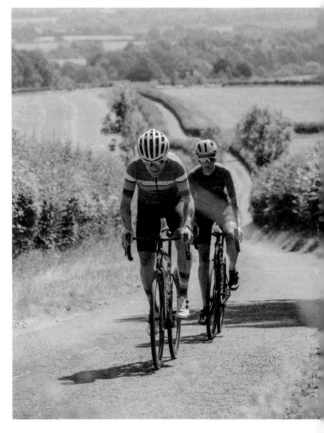

When it comes to climbing, your body weight is a key factor. As your power to weight ratio comes into play, those extra pounds can result in serious time losses over the hills.

How to use the nutritional labels

We are bombarded with enough data already as cyclists and, so you don't need to get bogged down in more numbers, I've put the meals and snacks into broader categories depending on their macronutrient and energy levels. You'll see these labels under the 'nutrition per serving' information in each recipe, telling you it's LOW-KCAL | LOW-CARB | LOW-PROTEIN or whatever it happens to be. This will make meal planning easy for you – choose a low-carb or lower energy meal or snack on rest days; a high-protein recipe when feeling sore or fatigued; and a high-carb or high-energy meal when you're planning an epic ride or adventure. Snack and main meals are classified slightly differently, so even though a high-carb snack can technically have fewer carbs than a low or medium carb main meal, it's the percentage of carbohydrate within the recipe that we're concerned with here. So, as I say, don't get caught up in the specific numbers, but use the macro categories as a guideline.

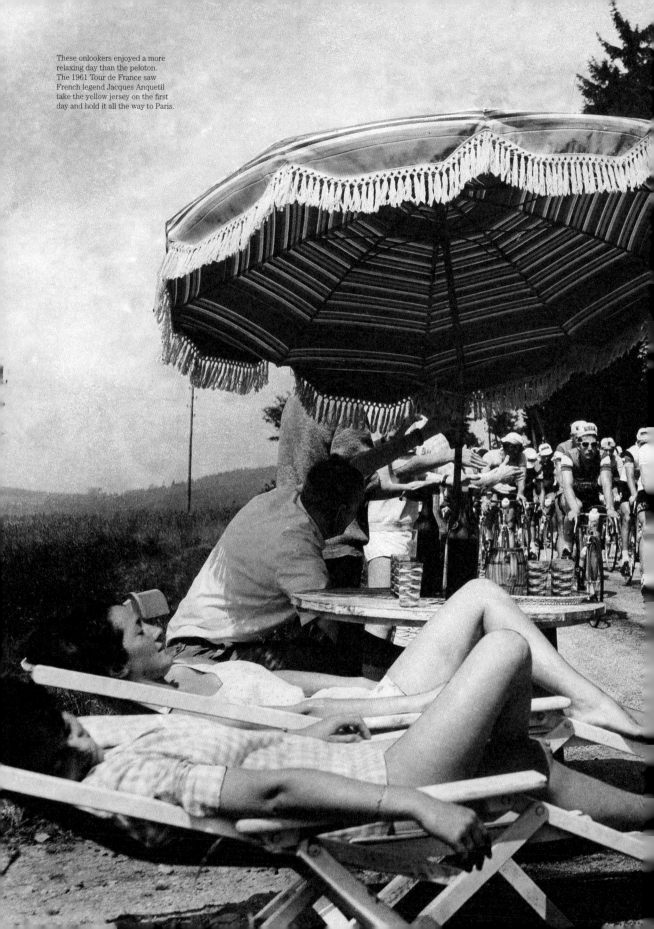

These onlookers enjoyed a more relaxing day than the peloton. The 1961 Tour de France saw French legend Jacques Anquetil take the yellow jersey on the first day and hold it all the way to Paris.

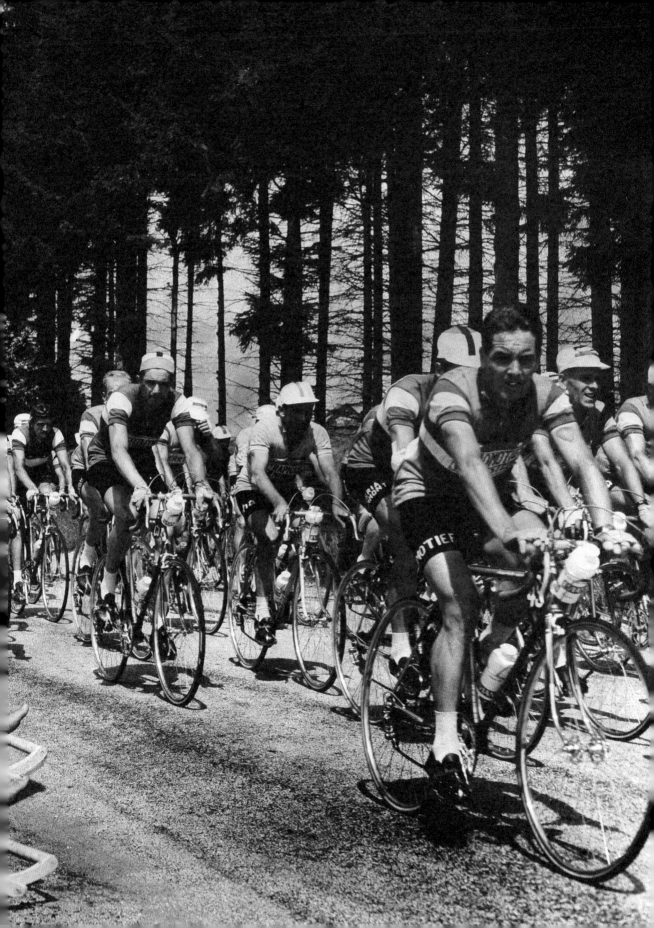

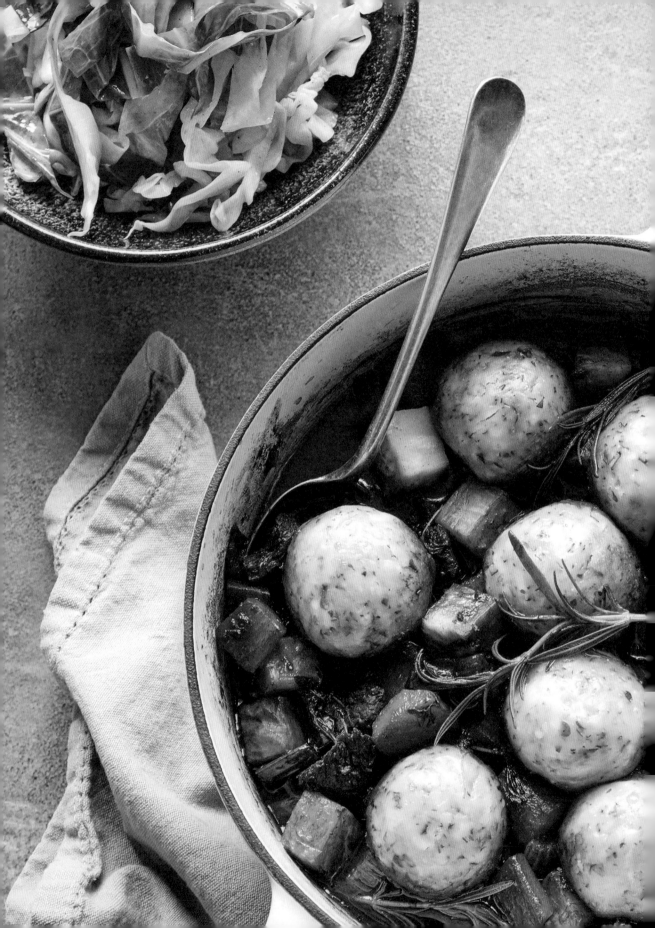

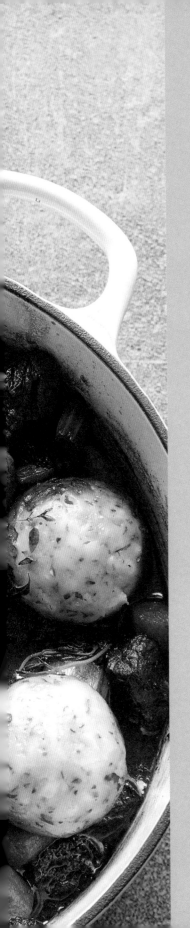

Off-season: Comforting winter warmers

The colder it is, the hungrier you'll probably feel, and during the off-season the natural impulse is to indulge. Gaining a couple of kilos at this time of year won't do you any harm. In fact, it may do you some good. However, during this period it's still important to resist the temptation to stuff yourself with endless treats and eat in proportion to how active you are. The recipes in this section, like my Asian pork with ginger and sesame (*see* p. 32), Boozy beef casserole with root veg, suet and thyme dumplings (*see* p. 38) or Creamy baked leeks with blue cheese and walnuts (*see* p. 36), are dense in nutrients, healthy and filling, so they'll satisfy that impulse to indulge, but won't lead to consistent overeating.

Murch's 'Not-tella' – mega-healthy chocolate, avocado and hazelnut spread

Here a classic, almost iconic, form of cyclist's fuel is given 'the treatment'. If you like your chocolate spread a little sweeter, add a touch more honey. The recipe can also be made suitable for our vegan friends by replacing the honey with maple syrup.

Makes 28 servings (20 g each)

25 g (1 oz) cocoa nibs

50 g (2 oz) hazelnuts, skin on

60 g (2½ oz) dates, pitted

180 g (6 oz) avocado flesh

40 g (1½ oz) cocoa powder

100 g (3½ oz) honey

100 ml (½ cup) water

pinch of sea salt

Nutrition per serving:
Energy: 53 kcal
Total carbohydrate: 5 g (of which sugars: 4.5 g)
Fat: 3.1 g (of which saturates: 0.8 g)
Fibre: 0.8 g | Protein: 1 g | Salt: 0.04 g

LOW-KCAL | LOW-CARB | LOW-PROTEIN

1. Place the cocoa nibs in the bowl of a food processor and blitz to a fine powder. Add the hazelnuts and repeat the process. Now add the dates and avocado, blitzing to a smooth paste.

2. Add the remaining ingredients and blend until smooth.

3. Transfer to an airtight container and refrigerate for up to 3 days.

French toast sandwich with smoked ham and grainy mustard

Like a posh toastie with egg… A simple and easy way to take the humble sandwich and elevate it. Works well with day-old bread and maybe serve with a spoon of my Kimchi (*see* p. 54). The overall calorie count can be brought down with thinner bread slices and by reducing the amount of cheese.

Serves 1

2 decent slices of sourdough

60 g (2½ oz) smoked ham, finely sliced

25 g (1 oz) mature cheddar

1 free-range egg, beaten

1 tablespoon milk

2 teaspoons grainy mustard

sea salt and freshly ground black pepper

10 g (½ oz) butter

green salad to serve

Nutrition per serving:
Energy: 801 kcal
Total carbohydrate: 83 g (of which sugars: 6 g)
Fat: 30 g (of which saturates: 14 g)
Fibre: 5.5 g | Protein: 46 g | Salt: 5.2 g

HIGH-KCAL | HIGH-CARB | HIGH-PROTEIN

1. First, make up your 'sandwich' of sourdough, ham, cheese, ham and then sourdough. Make sure the cheese is encased in the ham to ensure it won't melt out of the sandwich.

2. Use a fork to beat the egg in a bowl. Stir in the milk and mustard; season. Now pour the egg mix into a shallow dish and dip the sandwich in it, making sure both sides are well coated in the egg/mustard mix.

3. Melt the butter in a medium non-stick pan over a medium heat. Fry the sandwich for 2 minutes on each side until golden brown.

4. Remove from the pan, slice in half and arrange on a plate. Serve with green salad.

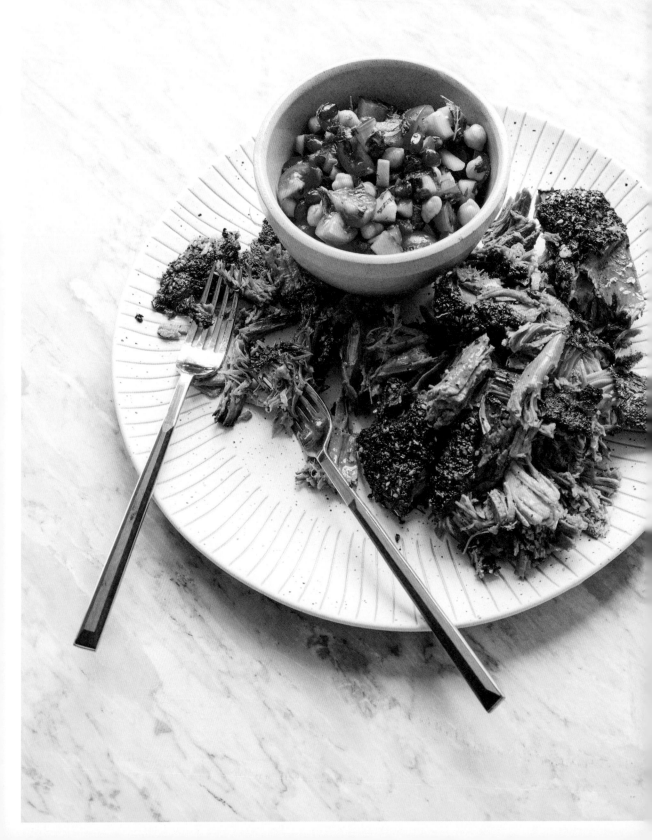

Za'atar roasted leg of lamb with pomegranate seeds, chickpeas and mint

Having worked in food for most of my life, it's rare to come across any revelations around ingredients but you never stop learning. My little sister Judy is a resident of New York City, which boasts arguably one of the world's most diverse food scenes. She introduced me to za'atar, an amazing herb/spice mixture of Middle Eastern origin with a truly stunning taste.

On a hungry day, serve with 200 g (7 oz) hummus and 4 large pitta breads (for 4 people, obviously). I would expect you all to have ridden your bikes for at least 3 hours if that's the case.

Serves 4

1 kg (2¼ lb) half a lamb leg joint with the bone in (about 500 g/1 lb 2 oz meat when cooked)

4 tablespoons za'atar

sea salt and freshly ground black pepper

Chickpea salsa

1 tin chickpeas (400 g/14 oz)

250 g (9 oz) pomegranate seeds

250 g (9 oz) fresh cherry tomatoes

1 cucumber, deseeded and diced

1 bunch of fresh mint, finely sliced

1 bunch of fresh coriander, chopped

1 teaspoon deseeded and diced green chilli

2 teaspoons fresh lemon juice

1 tablespoon extra virgin olive oil

1 teaspoon za'atar

1. Preheat the oven to 140°C/275°F/Gas 1. Meanwhile, place the lamb joint in a roasting tray and rub the meat with the za'atar. Place in the centre of the oven and cook for 3½–4 hours, regularly basting with the fat that renders down from the lamb leg.

2. For the last 30 minutes, turn the oven up to 220°C/425°F/Gas 7.

3. When you remove the lamb from the oven, wrap in tin foil and allow to rest for 30 minutes.

4. Then shred the lamb with a large fork and set aside, keeping warm.

5. While the lamb is roasting, mix all the ingredients for the chickpea salsa together in a bowl and season well.

6. Serve the shredded lamb on a platter with the salsa.

Nutrition per serving:
Energy: 811 kcal
Total carbohydrate: 20 g (of which sugars: 9.4 g)
Fat: 56 g (of which saturates: 25 g)
Fibre: 9 g | Protein: 52 g | Salt: 1.6 g

HIGH-KCAL | LOW-CARB | HIGH-PROTEIN

Asian pork with ginger and sesame

Slow cooking is perfect for cyclists as you can throw all the ingredients in and get yourself away out cycling, coming home to a ready-cooked meal. These strong aromatic flavours go together perfectly – beef or lamb would also work well.

Serves 2

2 tablespoons olive oil

400 g (14 oz) diced pork shoulder

1 red pepper, deseeded and diced

1 yellow pepper, deseeded diced

1 large onion, peeled and diced

50 g (2 oz) fresh ginger, peeled and finely diced

600 ml (2½ cups) chicken stock

40 ml (2 tablespoons) soy sauce

75 ml (4½ tablespoons) sweet chilli sauce

40 ml (2 tablespoons) Thai fish sauce

1 head pak choi, shredded

¼ head Chinese leaf or Savoy cabbage, finely sliced

small bunch of fresh coriander

1 teaspoon toasted sesame seeds

75 g (3 oz) white rice per person (dry-weight, cook according to the directions on the pack) to serve

Nutrition per serving:
Energy: 988 kcal
Total carbohydrate: 103 g (of which sugars: 38 g)
Fat: 37 g (of which saturates: 7.5 g)
Fibre: 11 g | Protein: 56 g | Salt: 9 g

HIGH-KCAL | HIGH-CARB | HIGH-PROTEIN

1. Heat half the olive oil in a large frying pan and brown the diced pork over a medium heat for 4–5 minutes before adding to the slow cooker.

2. Heat the remaining oil in the same pan and fry the peppers, onion and ginger for 3–4 minutes. Add to the slow cooker.

3. Add the stock, soy sauce, sweet chilli sauce and Thai fish sauce to the slow cooker, stirring to combine all the ingredients. Simmer over a low heat for 3 hours or until the meat is tender.

4. To finish, add the pak choi, cabbage and coriander and sprinkle over the sesame seeds. Serve with boiled rice.

Salmon fishcakes with caper and lemon dressing

Homemade fishcakes are so satisfying and easy to make. Also, they taste so much better than the shop-bought varieties. You can use pretty much any fresh fish you can find but make sure you use the right potato – if the mix is too wet, shaping the cakes will be a tricky affair.

Serves 2

400 g (14 oz) Desirée potatoes

10 g (½ oz) butter

sea salt and freshly ground black pepper

150 g (5 oz) skinless, boneless salmon fillet

1 teaspoon jerk seasoning

1 medium free-range egg, beaten

1 tablespoon gluten-free flour

2 spring onions, trimmed and finely chopped

small bunch of fresh dill, finely chopped

1 dessertspoon olive oil for cooking

large bowl of green salad and lemon wedges to serve

Dressing

zest and juice of 1 lemon

1 tablespoon chopped capers

2 tablespoons extra virgin olive oil

1 tablespoon water

Nutrition per serving:
Energy: 639 kcal
Total carbohydrate: 47 g (of which sugars: 5.2 g)
Fat: 36 g (of which saturates: 8 g)
Fibre: 8.5 g | Protein: 27 g | Salt: 0.8 g

HIGH-KCAL | MEDIUM-CARB | HIGH-PROTEIN

1. Boil the potatoes until softened (about 15–20 minutes) and then make a mash, adding the butter as you mash the potato flesh. Don't overwork the mixture or it will become too sticky. Season well with salt and pepper and set aside.

2. While your potatoes are cooking, preheat the grill to medium. Season the salmon fillet with jerk seasoning and grill for 6–8 minutes, turning, until cooked; allow to cool.

3. Make the fishcakes by flaking the salmon into a bowl and mixing with the potato, beaten egg, flour, spring onions and dill. If the mix is too wet, add a touch more flour. Mould into rounds with your hands to make four fishcakes.

4. Heat the olive oil in a non-stick frying pan and fry the fishcakes over a medium to low heat for 2–3 minutes each side until golden.

5. Make a salad dressing by mixing together in a bowl the lemon zest and juice with the capers, extra virgin olive oil and water. Season well and drizzle over the salad. Serve the fishcakes with the salad and lemon wedges.

'Bad boy' Bombay potatoes, tikka-spiced chicken thighs and wilted greens

An alternative take on a curry meal. The potatoes could easily be switched for cauliflower if you're looking for a lower-carb option.

Serves 4

1 kg (2¼ lb) skinless and boneless chicken thighs

3 teaspoons tikka spice

1 teaspoon turmeric

1 tablespoon caraway seeds

1 tablespoon olive oil

Bombay potatoes

750 g (1½ lb) new potatoes, skin-on

50 g (2 oz) unsalted butter

1 large onion, peeled and diced

1 tablespoon grated fresh ginger

1 tablespoon Madras curry powder

250 g (9 oz) pre-washed baby spinach leaves

small bunch of coriander

1 tablespoon black onion seeds

Nutrition per serving:
Energy: 791 kcal
Total carbohydrate: 36 g (of which sugars: 7.1 g)
Fat: 38 g (of which saturates: 14 g)
Fibre: 8.6 g | Protein: 71 g | Salt: 0.87 g

HIGH-KCAL | MEDIUM-CARB | HIGH-PROTEIN

1. Preheat the oven to 190°C/375°F/Gas 5. Meanwhile, trim any excess fat off the chicken thighs and arrange them in a shallow dish.

2. In a bowl, mix together the tikka spice, turmeric, caraway seeds and olive oil. Rub the mixture on to the chicken thighs, making sure they are well-coated. Cover and leave to marinate at room temperature for 15 minutes.

3. Place a large non-stick pan on the stove over a medium heat and fry the chicken thighs for 2–3 minutes each side until golden brown. Transfer to an ovenproof dish and bake for 12 minutes. Cover and keep warm.

4. While the chicken is baking, cut the potatoes in half and pre-cook for 8–10 minutes in boiling, salted water. Strain and set aside.

5. Place the butter, onion and ginger in a sauté pan and cook, stirring, over a low heat for 3–4 minutes. Stir in the curry powder and cook for a further 4 minutes. Add the potatoes and cook gently for 3 minutes more – you want the mixture to be quite dry.

6. Turn up the heat and add the spinach. Cook quickly for about 9 seconds, turning, and then sprinkle in the coriander and onion seeds.

7. Serve the Bombay potatoes with the tikka thighs.

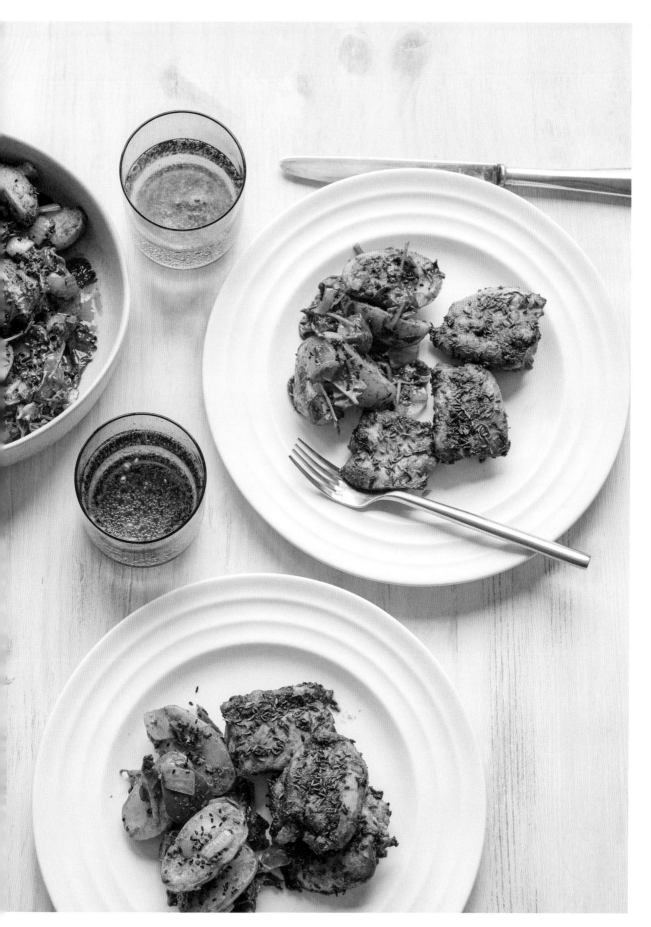

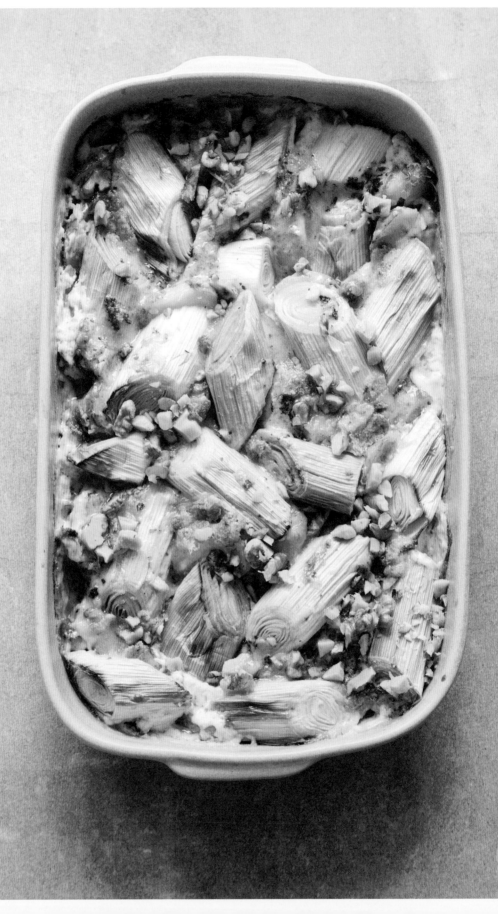

Creamy baked leeks with blue cheese and walnuts

A rich and decadent dish. Here leeks form the base of a cracking comfort dish as they have everything going for them, being tasty, cheap and widely available, yet they are rarely used outside of soups and broths. If blue cheese ain't your thing, replace with another strong cheese.

Serves 2

500 g (1 lb 2 oz) leeks, trimmed

25 g (1 oz) butter, melted

350 g (12 oz) cooked new potatoes, sliced

sea salt and freshly ground black pepper

150 ml (⅔ cup) single cream

pinch of grated nutmeg

90 g (3½ oz) Stilton

3 teaspoons chopped walnuts

green salad to serve

Nutrition per serving
Energy: 686 kcal
Total carbohydrate: 36 g (of which sugars: 12 g)
Fat: 48 g (of which saturates: 27 g)
Fibre: 11 g | Protein: 23 g | Salt: 1.3 g

HIGH-KCAL | MEDIUM-CARB | HIGH-PROTEIN

1. Preheat the oven to 160°C/325°F/Gas 3. Meanwhile, slice the leeks and wash thoroughly under cold running water. Drain well and pat dry on a clean tea towel.

2. Lightly brush the base of a 20 x 20 cm (8 x 8 in) ovenproof dish with melted butter.

3. Arrange the cooked potato slices in the base of the dish and season well.

4. In a bowl, combine the leeks with the single cream and nutmeg. Season well and pour over the potato base. Bake in the centre of the oven for 25 minutes, then sprinkle over the Stilton and walnuts. Return to the oven for a further 10 minutes.

5. Remove from the oven and allow to cool for 10 minutes, then serve with the green salad.

Boozy beef casserole with root veg, suet and thyme dumplings

Slow cooking for fast legs! This old-school cooking method is very much based around family meals we ate regularly when I was growing up, using less-fashionable cuts of meat and rustic root vegetables, which are big in flavour and low in cost. Perfect for a harder training day when calorie intake is less of an issue and also for time-crunched cyclists as it can be made up in advance and will keep for three to four days in the fridge. Dumplings are a great way of getting in extra carbs, but leave them out on low-carb days.

Serves 6

2 tablespoons olive oil

1 kg (2¼ lb) diced beef shoulder steak

200 g (7 oz) celery, trimmed and diced

200 g (7 oz) carrots, trimmed and diced

200 g (7 oz) celeriac, trimmed and diced

1 large onion, peeled and diced

600 ml (2½ cups) beef stock

400 ml (1½ cups) beer (local ale, not lager)

1 large sprig each of thyme and rosemary

fresh green vegetables to serve, such as broccoli, shredded cabbage and green beans

Dumplings (30 g/1¼ oz each)

150 g (5 oz) gluten-free self-raising flour

75 g (3 oz) beef suet

good pinch of salt

2 tablespoons finely chopped fresh thyme

8–10 tablespoons water

1. Place a large stockpot (with a lid available) over a high heat. Add the olive oil and then add the shoulder steak. Fry for 6–8 minutes until golden brown.

2. Add the diced vegetables and cook for a further 5 minutes. Stir in the beef stock, beer and herb sprigs.

3. Bring to the boil and simmer for 30 minutes, then put the lid on. Simmer for a further hour, remove from the heat and allow to rest for another hour.

4. While the casserole is simmering, make your dumplings. In a bowl, mix together the flour, suet, salt and thyme.

5. Add the water to form a firm but dry paste and shape with your hands to make the dumplings. Set aside until needed.

6. Once the casserole has rested, arrange the dumplings on top of the casserole, cover and simmer for 20 minutes. Remove the herb sprigs and serve with green vegetables.

Nutrition per serving:
Energy: 665 kcal
Total carbohydrate: 33 g (of which sugars: 7.1 g)
Fat: 29 g (of which saturates: 12 g)
Fibre: 3.9 g | Protein: 63 g | Salt: 1.6 g

HIGH-KCAL | MEDIUM-CARB | HIGH-PROTEIN

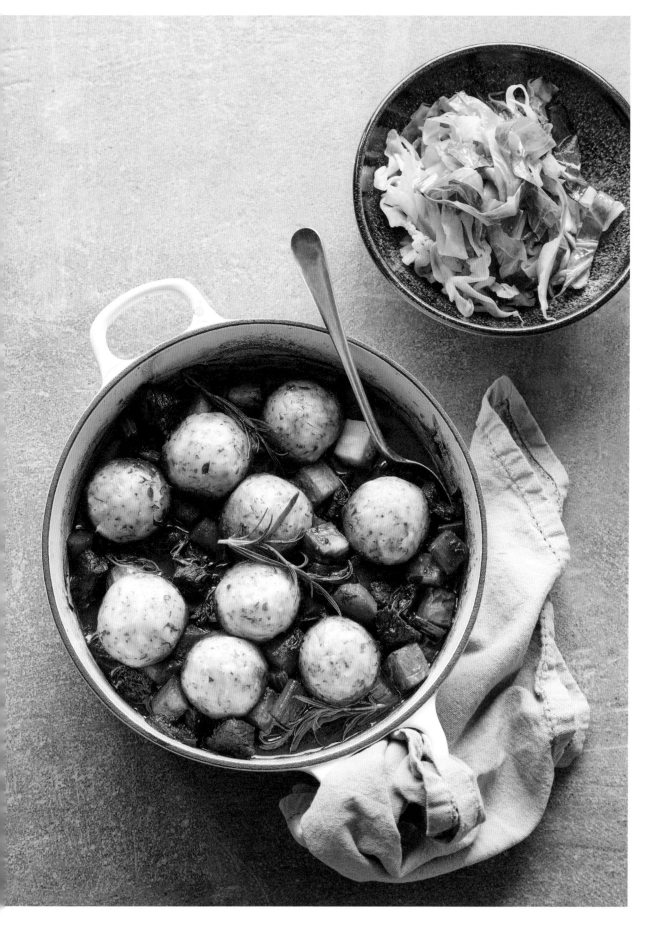

Baked chicken tortilla wraps with avocado salsa

A cracking wee recipe that can be made in advance and thrown in the oven when you get in from a ride. I reckon you have enough time to give your bike a quick clean, have a quick shower and the food will literally be on the table. For a lighter/lunch portion, serve one wrap per person with heaps of salad.

Serves 2

1 tablespoon olive oil for frying

2 small red onions, peeled and finely sliced

1 teaspoon chopped garlic

1 red pepper, deseeded and sliced

1 yellow pepper, deseeded and sliced

8 chicken mini fillets

3 teaspoons fajita spice

sea salt and ground black pepper

4 small tortilla wraps

butter for greasing

250 g (9 oz) passata

50 g (2 oz) grated cheddar

Salad

large pack of rocket salad

small bunch of coriander

1 medium avocado

1 small green chilli, deseeded and finely diced

juice of ½ a lime

1 teaspoon extra virgin olive oil

1. Preheat the oven to 180°C/350°F/Gas 4. Meanwhile, heat the olive oil in a large saucepan, add the onions and fry over a medium heat for 3–4 minutes

2. Add the garlic and peppers, cook for a further 3 minutes then add the chicken fillets and fajita spice. Cook slowly for 10 minutes, season well and allow to cool.

3. Divide the mix into four, spoon into the middle of the tortilla wraps and roll up carefully, tucking in the ends.

4. Lightly grease an ovenproof dish and arrange the tortilla wraps seamside down inside. Spoon over the passata, season and top with grated cheese. Bake in the centre of the oven for 20 minutes.

5. While the wraps are baking, make up a salad. Arrange the rocket salad and coriander leaves in a bowl. Remove the skin and stone from the avocado and roughly chop into the bowl. Add the chilli, lime juice and olive oil. Toss through and serve with the wraps.

Nutrition per serving:
Energy: 916 kcal
Total carbohydrate: 67 g (of which sugars: 25 g)
Fat: 39 g (of which saturates: 12 g)
Fibre: 14 g | Protein: 66 g | Salt: 3 g

HIGH-KCAL | MEDIUM-CARB | HIGH-PROTEIN

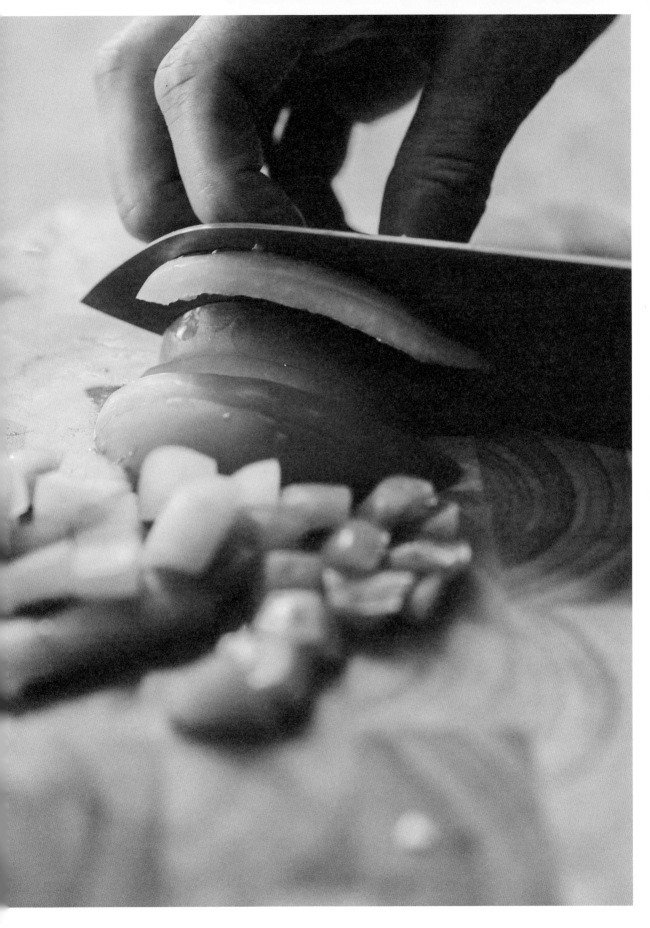

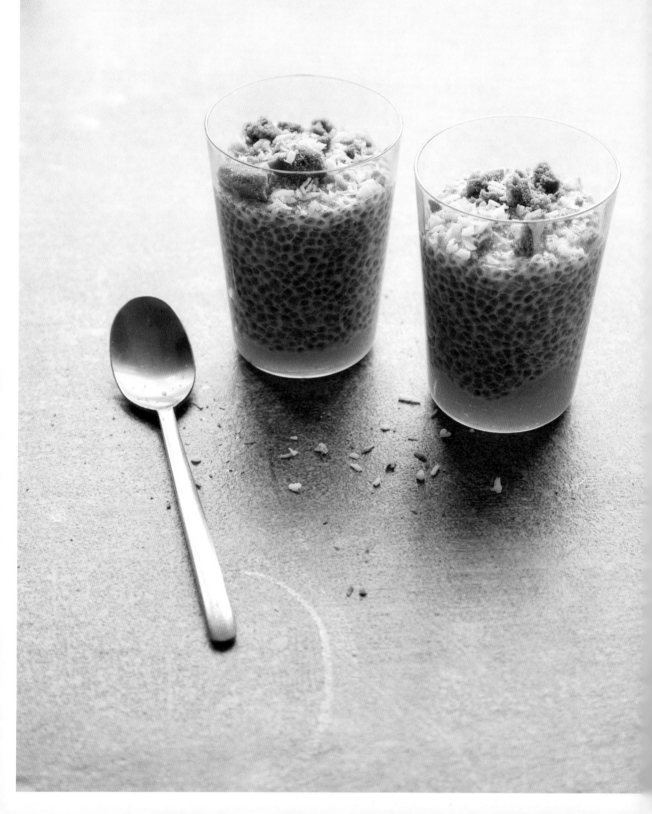

Coconut, lemon curd and gingerbread chia puddings

Now chia puddings can divide people… I love them, but I have heard comparisons with frog spawn in the past. This is such a simple method and you can save time by using shop-bought lemon curd and biscuits if you prefer. Raspberry jam as opposed to lemon curd would also work a treat. You can replace the coconut milk with unsweetened soya milk if you prefer – add a touch of honey to sweeten it.

Serves 4 (snack-size)

40 g (1½ oz) chia seeds

250 ml (1 cup) coconut milk (not the canned variety)

4 ginger nut biscuits

4 teaspoons lemon curd

1 tablespoon toasted desiccated coconut to serve

Nutrition per serving:
Energy: 191 kcal
Total carbohydrate: 22 g (of which sugars: 14 g)
Fat: 9 g (of which saturates: 4.2 g)
Fibre: 4.8 g | Protein: 2.9 g | Salt: 0.37 g

MEDIUM-KCAL | MEDIUM-CARB | LOW-PROTEIN

1. In a small jug, mix together the chia seeds and coconut milk. Cover and place in the fridge.

2. After 15 minutes, stir the mixture to ensure that it does not settle and separate.

3. Repeat this process a few times over 1½ hours then refrigerate for 3 hours.

4. Place the ginger nut biscuits in a clean plastic bag, seal and crush the biscuits with a rolling pin.

5. To assemble the puddings, spoon lemon curd into 4 small ramekins or glasses. Add the chia mix and then spoon over the crushed biscuits (hold back a small amount for serving).

6. Cover and refrigerate overnight. Just before serving, sprinkle each pudding with toasted coconut and the remaining crushed biscuit.

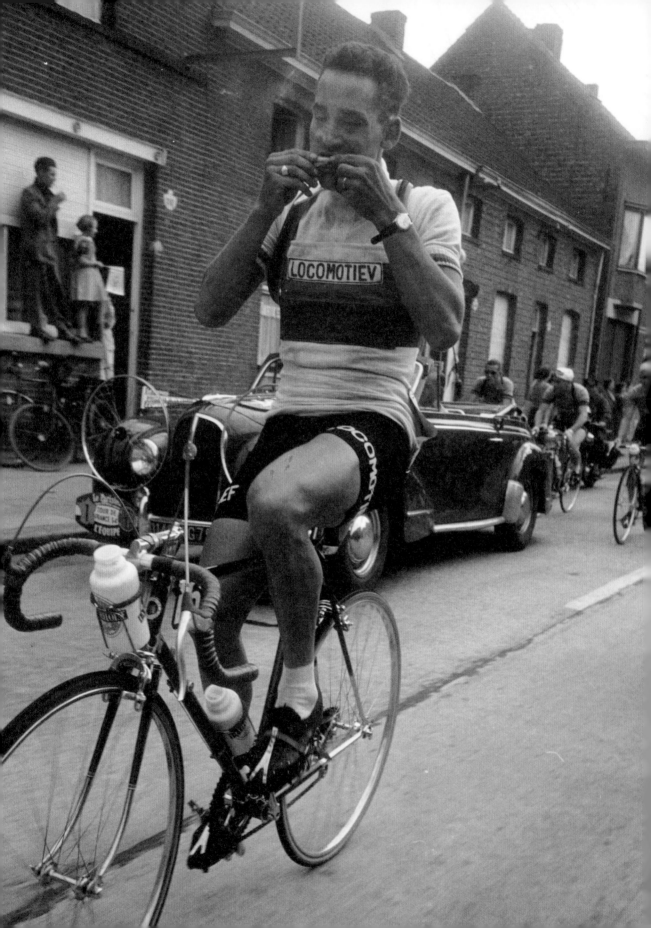

Eat Less,
Ride More

Are you a sprinter or a climber? Or are you a GC contender? Are you happy to be a club rider or do you have ambitions to challenge for national titles? Individual cyclists have different targets, but when it comes to weight loss everybody has exactly the same aim. The *British Medical Journal* spelt it out in a 2010 document that stated, 'Any intervention seeking to reduce body fat content must not only increase habitual physical activity, but also ensure that a negative energy balance is created by curtailing parallel increments of food intake.'[4] Forty years earlier, Eddy Merckx said much the same thing, but used fewer words, when the great Tour de France rider revealed his secret to losing weight: 'Eat less, ride more.'

Consuming calories on the go has always been a feature of cycling. But what and when you choose to eat has changed with the development of nutritional science.

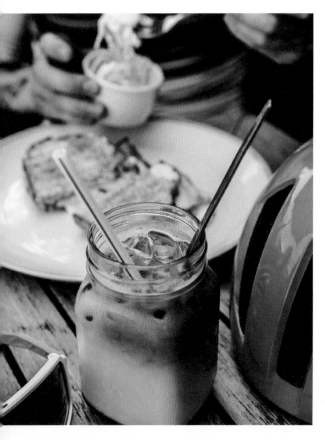

Breakfast is a crucial meal for cyclists. It's the perfect way to restore depleted muscle glycogen after a hard ride or to help deliver the energy required for a long day on the bike.

The word 'calories' is bandied about so frequently – in diets, on food packaging, even on the machine screens at the gym – that it's easy to forget exactly what they are. Calories are simply a measure of energy – no more, no less. They measure how much energy a foodstuff or a drink contains, or how much energy is expended by the body's life-sustaining organs, digestion or any physical activity, which means anything from sleeping to a 10-mile time trial. At the simplest level, to lose weight, you must consume fewer calories than you burn.

Once your body has used up all the available calories from the carbohydrates in your food, it turns to glycogen, the glucose stored in your muscles and liver. There's only a day or so's supply stowed there, so then it gets to work on your body fat, which contains around nine calories a gram and makes for a particularly rich source of energy. Only when those fat supplies become low will the amino acids within your muscles be broken down in a desperate scavenge for energy – and that's a situation any cyclist would definitely want to avoid.

A general rule of thumb is that your negative energy balance needs to be around 7000 calories (29,400 kilojoules) to lose one kilogram of fat. Cutting 350 calories a day from your diet should therefore enable you to lose a kilo in around 3 weeks. This is the same for men and women. My personal experience is that cutting out 500 calories a day over a 12-week period leads to a complete shift in my weight, although admittedly that's quite a challenging regime. If you do have one bad day, it's not the end of the world, but don't try to over-compensate on the following days – a 700–800 daily calorie deficit is too much and will have a negative impact.

Of course, it does depend on what your starting point is. You'll read in diet books that women should work from a baseline 2000 calories a day and men from 2500... unless you are an exceptional case. And cyclists *are* exceptional cases. Athletes' bodies might consume and expend energy in the same way as everyday folk, but their calorie consumption can be off the scale, with demands varying from day to day according to their training and racing schedules. Depending on your weight, speed and effort (gradient, head wind, etc.), you might burn through 400 to 1000 calories an hour. Over a week in which you put in two training rides and a race, you could be expending well over 5000 calories. Indeed, pro-cyclists in training or racing can work through 6000 or even 7000 calories a day.[5]

So far, so straightforward. You are burning through so many calories, it's easy to think it should be no problem to reduce your intake enough to lose weight quickly. However, Eddy Merckx was a great cyclist, but he was no nutritionist. The relationship between food and performance is a lot more complicated than he suggested. If anything, you need to monitor and control your food intake even more carefully than the sedentary office worker taking their crispbread and apple to work. Everything in our diet falls into three main food types (known as macronutrients) and each of them affects how well we ride our bikes.

Carbohydrates

Carbs are a combination of starch, sugars and fibre that are broken down to provide the body with energy. They come in two types, simple and complex. Simple carbs,

found in sweets, cakes and biscuits, are digested quickly and easily. Most diets will advise you to run a mile from such foods, but for endurance athletes they can provide a lightweight and efficient delivery of energy. On a ride over 90 minutes, cyclists will find energy bars, gels and drinks not only a useful, but an essential, provision.

Complex carbs deliver more sustained energy and are found in wholegrain pasta, bread, fruits, vegetables, beans and legumes. The body can store around 2000 calories of the sugars derived from carbs. These macronutrients are essential to cyclists and need to form around 50–60 per cent of daily calorie intake. Exactly how much carb-based food you require depends on the intensity of your training, but should range from around 5 to 10 grams a day per kilogram of body weight, so for reference 20 blueberries, one small apple or a breadstick contain about 15 grams of carbohydrate each.

Proteins

The amino acids that make up protein are the basic building blocks of the human body. For the cyclist, they are essential for the creation and repair of muscle tissue. Skimp on protein-rich foods such as eggs, lean meat, chicken, fish and nuts and you're going nowhere fast! Unlike carbs, the body doesn't store protein, so it needs to be included in most meals, as well as during, and especially after, a ride. The recommended protein intake for cyclists can easily be twice as high as for non-athletes, which can mean around 1.2 to

2 grams of protein per kilogram of body weight per day.[6] So, if you weigh 75 kg, that's up to 150 g of protein a day (and there's around 50 g of protein in a cooked chicken breast, no skin).

Fats

As fats contain more than twice the number of calories per gram as carbs or protein, you might be forgiven for thinking you should give them a wide berth. That's certainly true of the trans fats or hydrogenated fats which you find in crisps, biscuits and processed foods, but consumption of other fats is essential for health and performance. Among other benefits, they help the body absorb vitamins and play a vital role in muscle recovery. Saturated fats – found in butter and dairy products – should be consumed in moderation, but unsaturated fats, found in plants, nuts, lean meat and fish, should be an integral part of the cyclist's diet. Although it varies slightly depending on where you are in your training schedule, fats should make up around 25–30 per cent of your calories, which is more than enough to add flavour and interest.

The conundrum

The cyclist's body is a greedy creature with a voracious appetite. The muscles which drive it forward demand a deep and frequently replenished source of energy and a bountiful supply of nutrients and vitamins to enable them to grow and rejuvenate themselves. They want food and quite often they want it NOW! And you're going to cut down your calorie intake? That negative energy balance could so easily take a toll on your performance. You might find yourself losing power (remember the power

The cyclist's body is a greedy creature with a voracious appetite. Its muscles want food and quite often they want it NOW!

weight ratio, *see* pp. 16-17) or, even worse, suffering muscle depletion.

The good news is, of course, it can be done. Pro-cyclists manage their weight throughout the season, understanding when and by how much they can cut down to be in the right shape at the right time. If you're going to lose weight and maintain or even improve your times, you, too, are going to have to devise and stick to a dietary plan that suits your short- and long-term schedules. Here's a simple guide for balancing what you eat with your training load:

- Easy days: 40 per cent carbs + 30 per cent protein + 30 per cent fat
- Medium days: 50 per cent carbs + 30 per cent protein + 20 per cent fat
- Hard days: >60 per cent carbs + 30 per cent protein + 10 per cent fat
- Rest days: <25 per cent carbs + 50 per cent protein + 25 per cent fat[7]

Look, I'm a 49-year-old chef with a bad knee and pre-season I weighed 82 kg, but I got my weight down to 70 kg for race season and that took my metrics from good to excellent – in fact, it improved my metrics dramatically. Yes, you need attention to detail and discipline, but I'm living proof that it can be done.

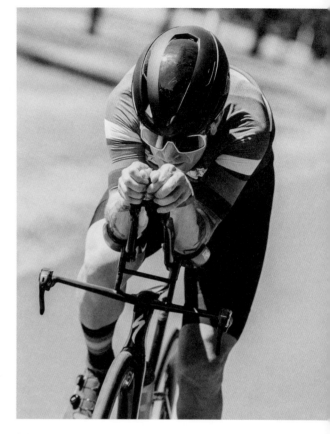

Fuelling correctly for your ride is essential. Riding full gas can burn through the calories and a negative energy balance could lead to you losing power.

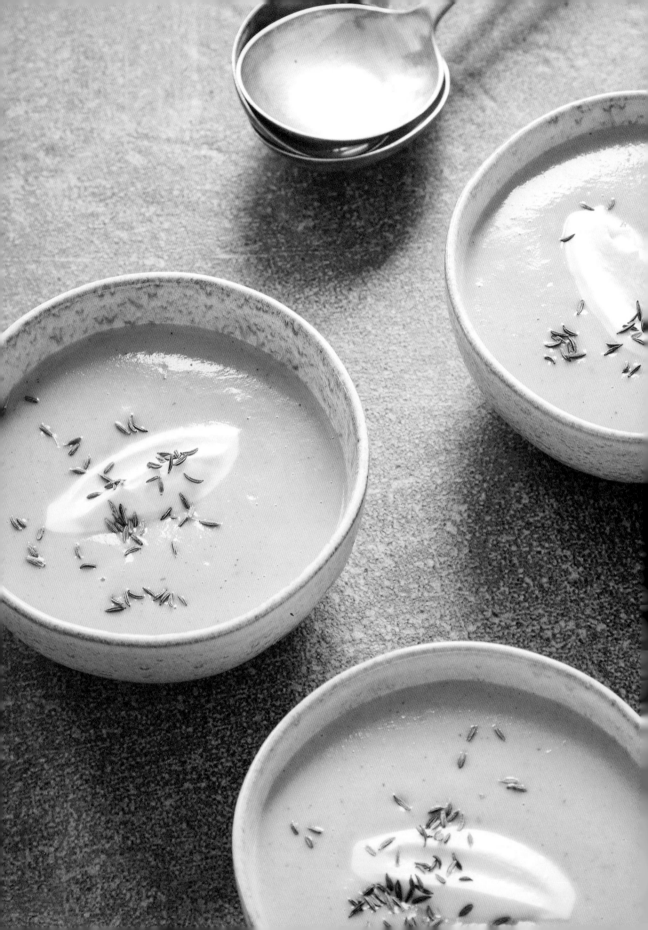

Pre-season: Lower carbs for body composition and getting back on track

Now's the time to start to get your training on track and your focus back, because what you do and eat pre-season is obviously going to affect your weight and your form once the season begins. So, cut down on carbs and up your intake of lean protein, fruit and veg to enhance the body's ability to burn fat for fuel. That doesn't mean your food has to be dull, though. Try my 'No-carb' easy-bake quiches with red onion and blue cheese (*see* p. 62) or Baked cod with tomato ketchup and tarragon relish (*see* p. 59) and my recipe for Kimchi (*see* p. 54) certainly delivers quite a kick!

Ginger-spiced granola with cinnamon and black pepper

Making your own granola is really simple to do. After making it for the first time, I promise you'll never buy it from the shops again! The granola will keep in an airtight container for up to 2 weeks.

Makes 12 portions (63 g/2.2 oz)

75 g (3 oz) honey

1 teaspoon freshly ground coarse black pepper

55 g (2¼ oz) coconut oil

75 g (3 oz) blackstrap molasses

250 g (9 oz) gluten-free oats

75 g (3 oz) desiccated coconut

75 g (3 oz) raisins

60 g (2½ oz) pumpkin seeds

60 g (2½ oz) sunflower seeds

4 teaspoons ground ginger

2 teaspoons ground cinnamon

pinch of sea salt

Greek yoghurt or milk of your choice to serve

Nutrition per serving (granola without yoghurt):
Energy: 287 kcal
Total carbohydrate: 30 g (of which sugars: 14 g)
Fat: 15 g (of which saturates: 8.3 g)
Fibre: 4.5 g | Protein: 6 g | Salt: 0.24 g

LOW-KCAL | LOW-CARB | LOW-PROTEIN

1. Preheat the oven to 140°C/275°F/Gas 1. Meanwhile, line a baking tray with greaseproof paper.
2. Place the honey, black pepper, coconut oil and molasses in a small pan. Melt over a gentle heat on the hob, stirring to combine.
3. Weigh out your dry ingredients into a large bowl. Pour in the molasses mixture and stir to combine thoroughly.
4. Transfer to the baking tray and smooth with a palette knife to spread out evenly. Bake in the centre of the oven for 45 minutes, gently mixing with a fork every 15 minutes. The granola will be sticky at first when it comes out of the oven but will cool to a nice crispiness.
5. Serve with a good dollop of Greek yoghurt or milk of your choice.

Easy tomato and basil soup

Medium-day soup… have yourself a chunk of bread to mop out the soup bowl afterwards.
A recipe with few ingredients, but so much flavour – and much better than tomato soup
from a tin!

Serves 4

50 g (2 oz) butter

2 onions, peeled and finely chopped

4 garlic cloves, peeled and crushed

1 heaped tablespoon plain flour

750 ml (3 cups) vegetable stock

3 tins (400 g/14 oz) chopped tomatoes

60 g (2½ oz) runny honey

100 ml (½ cup) white wine vinegar

sea salt and ground black pepper

small bunch of chopped basil

Nutrition per serving:
Energy: 297 kcal
Total carbohydrate: 36 g (of which sugars: 25 g)
Fat: 13 g (of which saturates: 7.6 g)
Fibre: 5.1 g | Protein: 5.6 g | Salt: 2 g

LOW-KCAL | MEDIUM-CARB | LOW-PROTEIN

1. Place the butter in a large soup pan and melt over a low heat. Add the onions and garlic and fry gently for 4–5 minutes until translucent.

2. Add the flour and stir into the onion mix. Cook over a low heat, stirring, for 3 minutes.

3. Gradually stir in the vegetable stock, then add the chopped tomatoes. Simmer for 25–30 minutes, stirring every so often to ensure the bottom of the pan doesn't catch. Remove from the heat and allow to cool for 20 minutes, then liquidise. Set aside.

4. Now make what we in the trade call a gastric – basically a sweet and acid mix. Put your honey in a pan and boil for 2 minutes, stirring occasionally, then add the white wine vinegar and boil for a further minute. Pour this mix into the tomato base and adjust the seasoning.

5. Transfer the soup to bowls and finish off with some chopped fresh basil to serve.

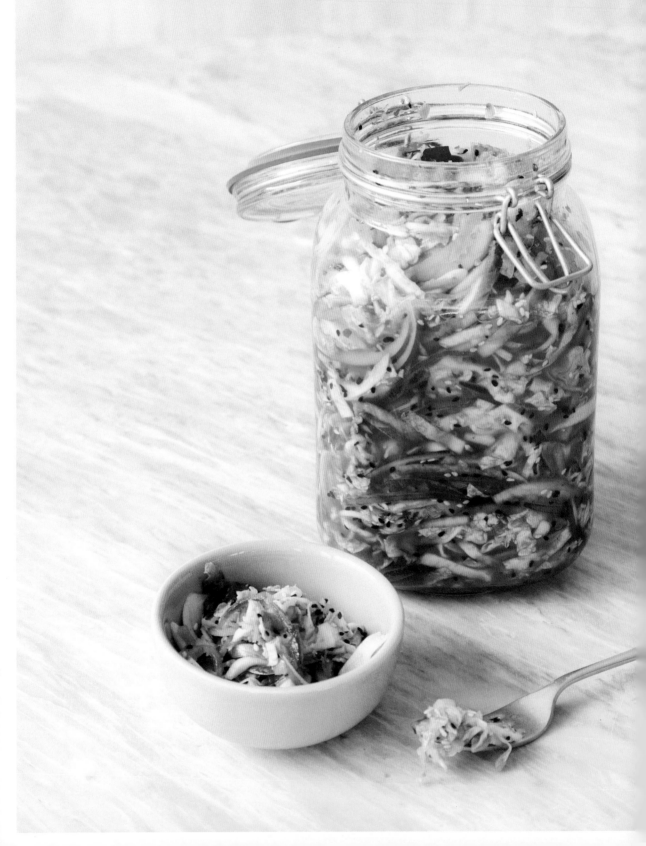

Kimchi by Murchi

An easy take on a fermented hipster cabbage dish. Fermented dishes are hugely beneficial for gut bacteria, which is the basis of good health according to many an expert. I think it tastes nice and is basically a great way of using up an old cabbage! The nutritional info here is for a portion of the Kimchi. However, it's also perfect served up with cooked rice (75 g/3 oz uncooked weight) and a couple of fried eggs for a simple, tasty meal. Sweet, salty, sour, crunchy and oh, so cheap!

Makes quite a lot (24 x 55 g/2¼ oz servings)

1 large cabbage (about 700 g/1 lb 7 oz)

3 teaspoons pink Himalayan salt

2 large carrots, trimmed, peeled and grated

1 red onion, peeled and finely sliced

60 g (2½ oz) fresh ginger, peeled and finely chopped

2 tablespoons Thai fish sauce

2 teaspoons black sesame seeds

2 teaspoons white sesame seeds

2 tablespoons chilli sauce

5 garlic cloves, peeled, crushed and sliced

1 tablespoon brown sugar

3 tablespoons rice or white wine vinegar

Nutrition per serving (per 55 g/2¼ oz serving):
Energy: 31 kcal
Total carbohydrate: 4.6 g (of which sugars: 4.1 g)
Fat: 0.5 g (of which saturates: 0 g)
Fibre: 1.6 g | Protein: 1 g | Salt: 1 g

LOW-KCAL | LOW-CARB | LOW-PROTEIN

1. Trim and slice up your cabbage. Place in a large bowl. Add the salt and combine with your hands. Allow to sit for 1 hour.

2. Mix together the carrots and onion in another bowl and set aside.

3. Make a wet paste with the remaining ingredients in another bowl.

4. Rinse the salt from the cabbage and pat dry on a clean tea towel. Combine all ingredients together in a bowl and transfer to a sterilised jar (see box below), pressing it down with your hands.

5. Leave overnight at room temperature and refrigerate for a minimum of 48 hours. The mixture will keep in the fridge for up to 4 weeks.

Sterilising the jar

Preheat the oven to medium (180°C/350°F/Gas 4). Meanwhile, wash the jar and lid in warm, soapy water. Rinse well, then dry thoroughly with a clean tea towel. Place the jar on a roasting tray and pop in the oven for 5 minutes.

Spicy roast parsnip soup with cumin and caraway

Medium-calorie... it's worth having a good chunk of bread with this easy-to-make soup if you're pushing on! It can be made using any manner of root veg – literally, whatever you find in the bottom of the fridge. The soup freezes really well. Allow leftover soup to cool and then pop into a suitably sized airtight container or it can be handy frozen in individual portions for quick and easy lunches. It keeps in the freezer for 4–6 weeks. When reheating, it's important to do this over a low heat as it will burn quite easily.

Makes 6 portions

100 g (3½ oz) unsalted butter

1 medium onion, peeled and diced

600 g (1¼ lb) parsnips, peeled and diced

1 teaspoon turmeric

3 teaspoons tikka curry powder

1500 ml (3 pints) vegetable stock

500 ml (2 cups) semi-skimmed milk

sea salt and ground black pepper

1 teaspoon low-fat crème fraîche per person to serve

1 teaspoon cumin seeds to serve

1 teaspoon caraway seeds to serve

Nutrition per serving:
Energy: 319 kcal
Total carbohydrate: 21 g (of which sugars: 12 g)
Fat: 22 g (of which saturates: 14 g)
Fibre: 5.6 g | Protein: 6 g | Salt: 1.9 g

LOW-KCAL | LOW-CARB | LOW-PROTEIN

1. Melt the butter in a large soup pan and fry the onion over a low heat for 3–4 minutes until softened.

2. Add the parsnips and turn up the heat. Over a medium heat, cook the parsnip mix for 5 minutes until slightly coloured.

3. Stir the turmeric and tikka curry powder into the pan and cook for a further 2 minutes.

4. Add the stock and milk and simmer for 30 minutes until the parsnips are tender. Remove from the heat and allow to cool for 15 minutes before liquidising until smooth and then adjust the seasoning.

5. Serve in bowls with a dollop (teaspoon) of crème fraîche on each one and sprinkle over some cumin and caraway seeds.

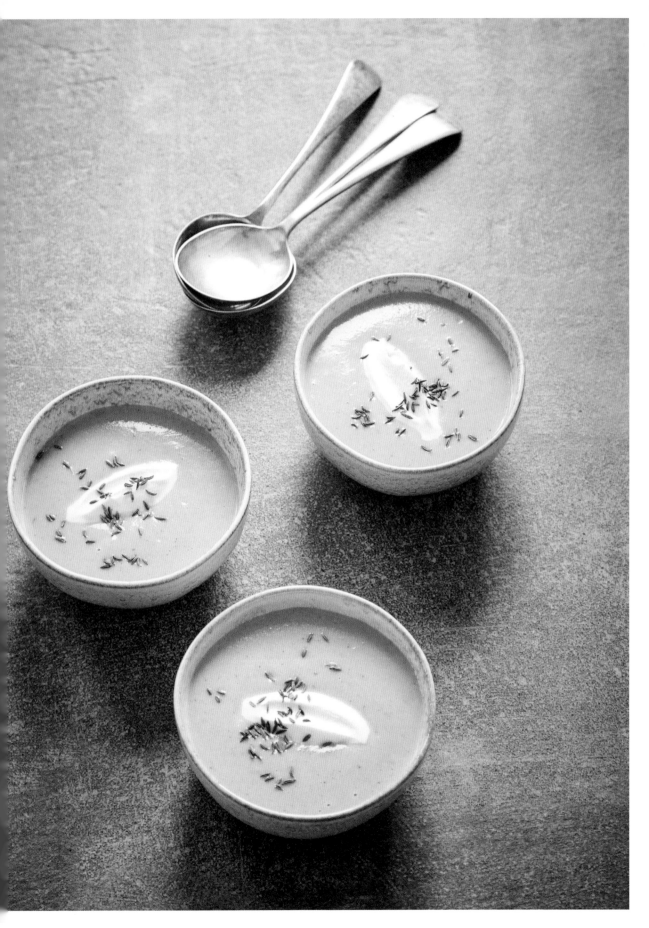

Thai-style beef and raw vegetable salad

Ideal for a rest day vibe, this raw veg salad with Thai influences has great texture and flavour and goes well with flash-fried steak. If you're looking to make this dish more carby, add 50 g (2 oz) rice noodles (dry-weight per person) dressed with a tablespoon of sweet chilli sauce per portion.

Serves 2

2 teaspoons olive oil

300 g (11 oz) minute steak

sea salt and freshly ground black pepper

Raw vegetable salad

4 teaspoons roughly chopped coriander

1 red onion, peeled and sliced

½ red pepper, deseeded and sliced

½ yellow pepper, deseeded and sliced

250 g (9 oz) beansprouts

2 tablespoons soy sauce

2 tablespoons Thai fish sauce

2 teaspoons black sesame seeds, toasted if liked

2 teaspoons white sesame seeds, toasted if liked

30 g (1¼ oz) grated fresh ginger

1. Prepare your raw vegetable salad as the first job. In a bowl, mix together the coriander, onion and peppers with the beansprouts.

2. Stir in the soy sauce, Thai fish sauce, half of the black and white sesame seeds and the ginger. Cover and set aside for 10 minutes to marinate.

3. Set a medium grill pan over a high heat and once heated, add the olive oil. Fry the steak very quickly for 20 seconds each side. Remove from the pan, season well and allow to rest on a warmed plate for 5 minutes.

4. Once the steak has rested, slice finely. Arrange the slices over the top of the salad. Spoon over the juices from the steak and serve finished off with the remaining sesame seeds.

Nutrition per serving:
Energy: 389 kcal
Total carbohydrate: 19 g (of which sugars: 13 g)
Fat: 15 g (of which saturates: 3.3 g)
Fibre: 5.8 g | Protein: 43 g | Salt: 6.4 g

LOW-KCAL | LOW-CARB | HIGH-PROTEIN

Baked cod with tomato ketchup and tarragon relish

A Michelin-starred chef using tomato ketchup? Whatever next! This is a simple, light dish. You can make up a double portion of relish as it keeps really well in the fridge for up to a week. The relish also works very well with grilled meats or on a big bacon sandwich.

Serves 2

1 teaspoon olive oil

2 x 150 g (5 oz) cod fillets

200 g (7 oz) French beans, trimmed

2 teaspoons fresh lemon juice

500 g (1 lb 2 oz) new potatoes, peeled, cooked, sliced and set aside in a large bowl

Tomato ketchup and tarragon relish

100 g (3½ oz) tomato ketchup

1 tablespoon Dijon mustard

1 tablespoon extra virgin olive oil

1 teaspoon white wine vinegar

small red onion, peeled and finely chopped

small bunch of tarragon, about 2 chopped tablespoons' worth

1. Preheat the oven to 190°C/375°F/Gas 5. Meanwhile, spoon the olive oil on to a plate, roll the cod fillets in it and arrange on a non-stick baking tray. Bake in the centre of the oven for 10–12 minutes.

2. Make the relish by whisking all the ingredients together in a bowl and set aside.

3. To bring everything together, simmer the French beans in boiling salted water for 3–4 minutes while the cod is cooking. Sprinkle the lemon juice over the cod, then pour the cooking juices from the fish over the sliced potatoes. Serve the potatoes cold with the fish, beans and the relish.

Nutrition per serving:
Energy: 488 kcal
Total carbohydrate: 57 g (of which sugars: 20 g)
Fat: 11 g (of which saturates: 1.7 g)
Fibre: 8.8 g | Protein: 35 g | Salt: 2 g

MEDIUM-KCAL | MEDIUM-CARB | HIGH-PROTEIN

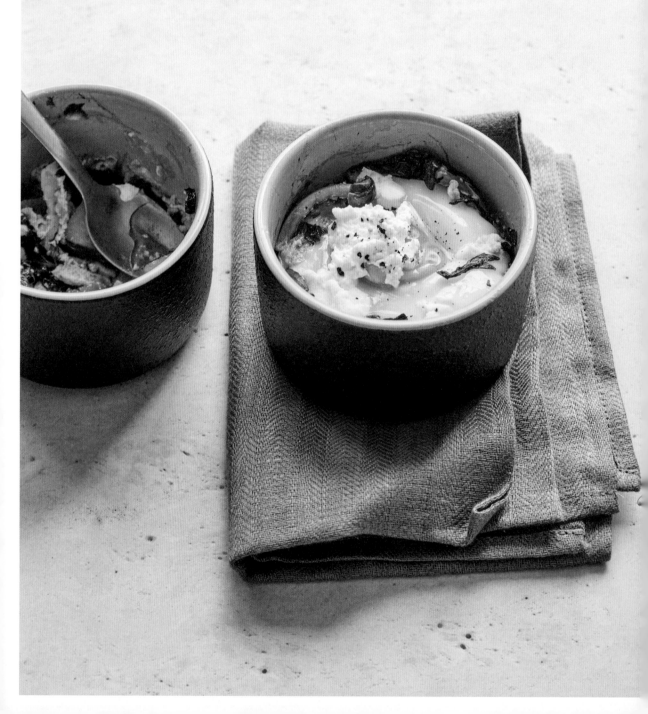

Baked duck eggs with spinach, ricotta and wild mushrooms

As standard, this is low-carb and high-protein. Full-fat dairy also means it will make you feel nice and full – great when you're on a low-carb day. Duck eggs are now widely available and have a pretty unique flavour. Usually larger than hen eggs, they are higher in magnesium, calcium, iron and B12. They also have more calories, which can be a good thing. This 'cracking' dish (see what I did there!) can be carbed up by serving with toasted chunks of bread.

Makes 2 or 4 portions (2 eggs per person as a main meal or 1 egg for a light lunch)

2 x 25 g (1 oz) butter

250 g (9 oz) baby spinach leaves

sea salt and freshly ground black pepper

250 g (9 oz) mixed mushrooms (shiitake, oyster, chestnut), chopped

2 teaspoons chopped garlic

100 g (3½ oz) ricotta cheese

4 free-range duck eggs

Nutrition per serving:
Energy: 345 kcal
Total carbohydrate: 4.4 g (of which sugars: 1.7 g)
Fat: 26 g (of which saturates: 13 g)
Fibre: 1.6 g | Protein: 22 g | Salt: 1.4 g

Snack version:
LOW-KCAL | LOW-CARB | HIGH-PROTEIN

Main meal:
MEDIUM-KCAL | LOW-CARB | HIGH-PROTEIN

1. Preheat the oven to 190°C/375°F/Gas 5. Melt half the butter in a large sauté pan, add the spinach and fry for 2–3 minutes until wilted down. Season well, then transfer to a colander. Press out any excess liquid with your fingertips and set aside in a bowl.

2. Now add the remaining butter to the same pan (there's no need to wash the pan). Add the mushrooms and garlic and fry over a medium heat for 4–5 minutes until the mushrooms are golden brown. Season and transfer to the colander to drain off any excess juices. Allow to cool.

3. Take 4 large ramekins and spoon in the garlic mushrooms evenly. Now add the spinach and make a small indentation or 'nest' with your fingertip.

4. Add a teaspoon of ricotta to the spinach, then crack a duck egg into each ramekin. Top off with the remaining ricotta and season.

5. Arrange the ramekins on a baking tray and bake in the centre of the oven for 12 minutes or until the egg whites are cooked and the yolks are still a bit runny.

'No-carb' easy-bake quiches with red onion and blue cheese

High-protein, perfect after a short, hard ride, these low-carb quiches can easily be made up in advance. Use this basic recipe to freestyle and design your own favourites. Cured ham, smoked salmon, edamame beans, peas, spinach… Anything else knocking about? Any fresh herbs you have in the fridge can be added to the mix for extra flavour – soft herbs like parsley and dill work particularly well.

Makes 2–3 'quiches' depending on the size of ramekin or one portion

3 large free-range eggs

3 tablespoons semi-skimmed milk

sea salt and freshly ground black pepper

1 tablespoon chopped fresh herbs (your choice)

2 teaspoons olive oil

1 small red onion, peeled and finely sliced

1 teaspoon sherry or balsamic vinegar

a little soft butter for greasing the ramekins

30 g (1¼ oz) Stilton or Roquefort cheese, cut into small chunks

1. Preheat the oven to 180°C/350°F/Gas 4. Meanwhile, in a bowl, whisk together the eggs and milk. Season well, stir in any fresh herbs you fancy and set aside.

2. Heat the olive oil and fry the onion over a low heat for 8–10 minutes until softened. Add the vinegar and cook out until the mixture becomes sticky. Once cool, stir the onion mixture into the eggs.

3. Take 2 medium ramekins and grease with butter, ensuring an even coating. Fill the ramekins with the egg mixture and top with cheese.

4. Bake in the centre of the oven for 15 minutes, then allow to cool for 5 minutes before turning out on to plates.

Nutrition per serving:
Energy: 513 kcal
Total carbohydrate: 12 g (of which sugars: 8.8 g)
Fat: 36 g (of which saturates: 13 g)
Fibre: 4 g | Protein: 33 g | Salt: 1.4 g

MEDIUM-KCAL | LOW-CARB | HIGH-PROTEIN

Grilled salmon with beetroot, chia, kidney bean and red onion salsa

Carbs and protein, ready to eat in under 10 minutes. This is probably one of the quickest meals you will ever make: simply grill fish and open a can, measure out a few store-cupboard staples... Simples!

Serves 2

2 x 130 g (4¼ oz) salmon fillets per person

1 teaspoon olive oil for cooking

sea salt and freshly ground black pepper

juice of ½ lemon to serve

bag of rocket salad to serve

Salsa

juice of 1 lemon

1 tin (400 g/14 oz) kidney beans in water

300 g (11 oz) cooked, diced beetroot

1 small red onion, peeled and finely chopped

1 red pepper, deseeded and finely chopped

2 tablespoons sweet chilli sauce

1 tablespoon extra virgin olive oil

1 teaspoon sherry vinegar

3 teaspoons chia seeds

1. Preheat the grill, nice and hot. Place the salmon fillets on a non-stick baking sheet, coat in oil and season well. Grill for 6–8 minutes, turning once.

2. While the salmon is cooking, make the salsa: simply combine all the ingredients together in a bowl. Check the seasoning and set aside.

3. When the salmon is cooked, add a good squeeze of lemon juice and serve with the salsa and rocket leaves.

Nutrition per serving:
Energy: 711 kcal
Total carbohydrate: 53 g (of which sugars: 32 g)
Fat: 32 g (of which saturates: 5.2 g)
Fibre: 19 g | Protein: 42 g | Salt: 0.29 g

HIGH-KCAL | MEDIUM-CARB | HIGH-PROTEIN

Watermelon, feta and Serrano ham salad

Light, crisp and refreshing, this is a perfect rest day meal. If you are feeling fancy, use different varieties of melon. You can also quite easily carb this bad boy up with the addition of some roasted chunks of sweet potato.

Serves 2

6 slices Serrano or Parma ham (3 per person)

400 g (14 oz) watermelon, diced

150 g (5 oz) feta cheese, diced

small bag of rocket salad

50 g (2 oz) walnuts

Dressing

1 teaspoon runny honey

1 tablespoon extra virgin olive oil

1 teaspoon white wine vinegar

Nutrition per serving:
Energy: 586 kcal
Total carbohydrate: 19 g (of which sugars: 18 g)
Fat: 42 g (of which saturates: 14 g)
Fibre: 1.9 g | Protein: 31 g | Salt: 1.9 g

MEDIUM-KCAL | LOW-CARB | HIGH-PROTEIN

1. Shred the ham with your fingertips. Combine with the watermelon and feta in a serving bowl.
2. In another bowl, mix together the honey, olive oil and white wine vinegar.
3. Combine the watermelon mix with the rocket salad and sprinkle over the walnuts.
4. Spoon over the honey dressing and get stuck in!

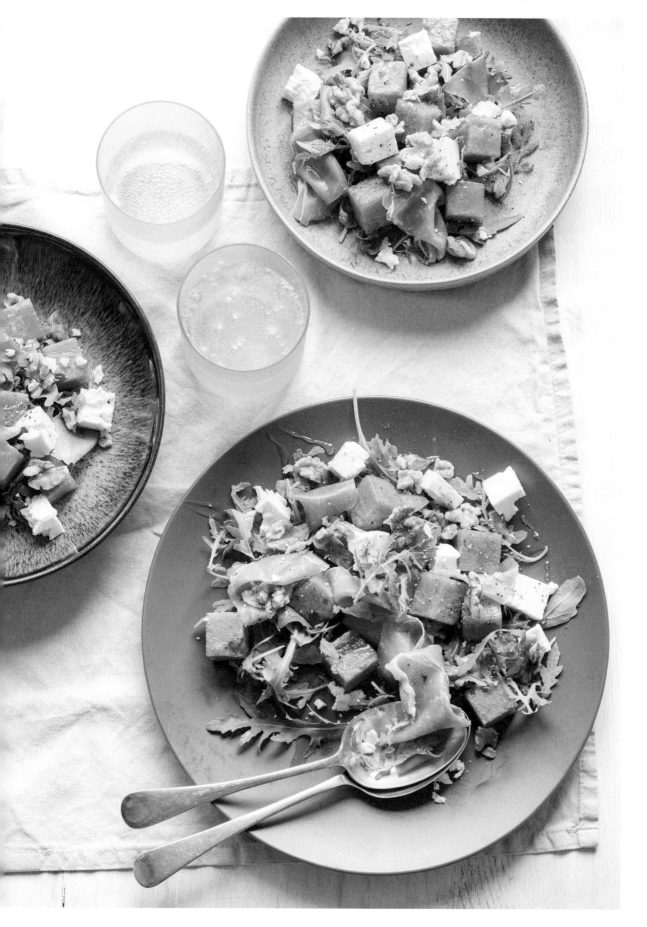

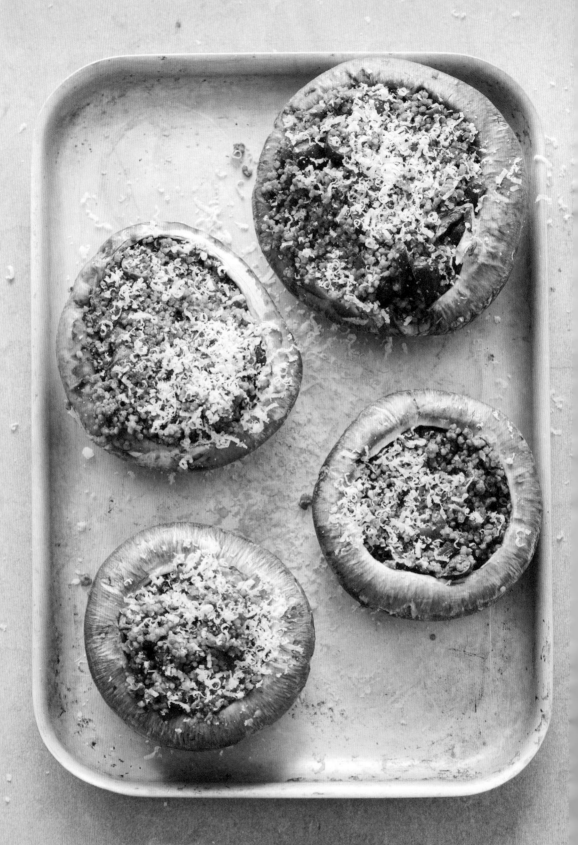

Baked portobello mushrooms, kale and quinoa pesto

Please read on as normally when you mention kale and quinoa in the same sentence people turn the page. This is a cracking way of getting in your greens and carbs in one simple hit. The kale pesto can be made up in advance and keeps in the fridge for 5 days. This works well with a number of grains, including freekeh, bulgur wheat and couscous. For fewer calories, take the portion down to one mushroom per person.

Serves 4

8 large portobello or field mushrooms, up to 10 cm (4 in) across

1 teaspoon olive oil for cooking

sea salt and freshly ground black pepper

50 g (2 oz) black olives, pitted

40 g (1½ oz) green olives, pitted

40 g (1½ oz) tahini

400 g (14 oz) cooked quinoa

4 teaspoons grated Parmesan or hard vegan cheese, if you are that way inclined

Pesto

300 g (11 oz) kale

200 g (7 oz) Brazil nuts

100 ml (½ cup) extra virgin olive oil

100 ml (½ cup) water

zest of 2 lemons

1. Preheat the oven to 150°C/300°F/Gas 2. Meanwhile, remove the stalks from the mushrooms and brush the cups with olive oil. Season well and set aside.

2. Make the pesto by blending the kale, Brazil nuts, olive oil, water and lemon zest until you have a smooth paste.

3. Chop the olives and transfer to a bowl. Stir in the tahini and quinoa, then stir in 1 tablespoon of pesto per portion (so, 4 tablespoons altogether) until you have a nice sticky mix. Check the seasoning.

4. Spoon the quinoa mix into the mushroom cups and press firmly with your fingertips. Top with cheese and transfer to an ovenproof dish. Bake in the centre of the oven for 10 minutes until golden and bubbling.

Nutrition per serving:
Energy: 886 kcal
Total carbohydrate: 25 g (of which sugars: 8.7 g)
Fat: 73 g (of which saturates: 15 g)
Fibre: 13 g | Protein: 26 g | Salt: 1.2 g

HIGH-KCAL | LOW-CARB | HIGH-PROTEIN

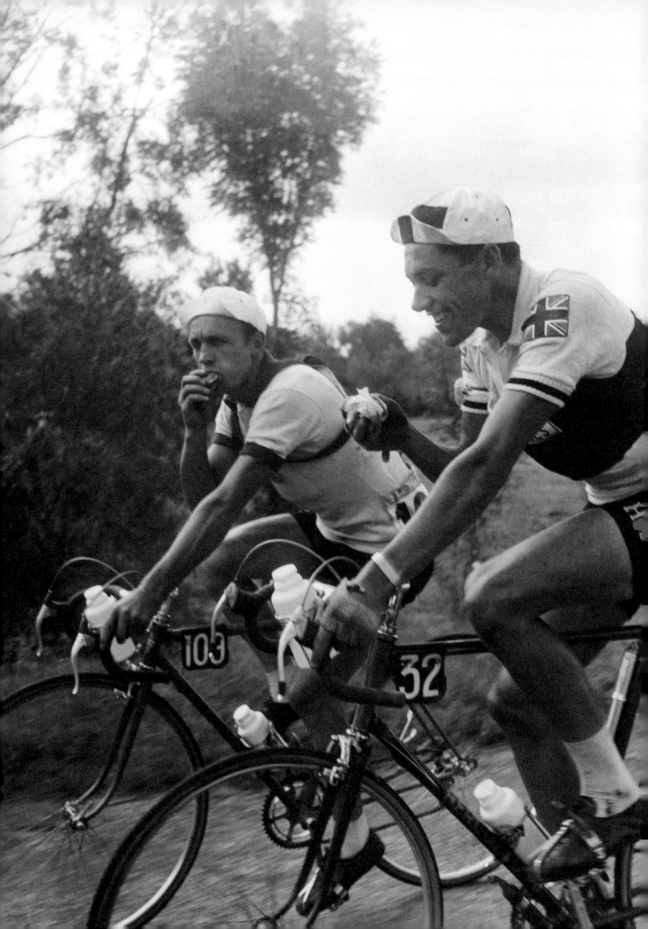

So Many Diets…

Eating is a deeply pleasurable experience. That's not me writing as a chef or even as a guy who likes his food, it's a scientific fact. Neuroscientists have established that eating is not only essential to survival, it is also one of our main routes to pleasure[8] – whether that's through the multi-sensual properties of food, the process of feeding yourself or the memories and other associations it carries. To deny yourself the pleasure of eating makes no sense and any diet that ignores the pleasure principle is sooner or later doomed to failure, so rule number one is always enjoy your food.

Some fad diets can take such a grip on the public imagination that even someone like myself, who instantly recoils from them, has heard of the Atkins Diet, the Paleo Diet, the 5:2 Diet and the Keto Diet. These diets are well known for a reason: they work. They work because, no matter how they are dressed up and marketed, they basically follow the negative energy balance principle – calories expended exceed calories

Claude Colette (left) and Tony Hoar (right) refuel during the 1955 Tour de France. Hoar later won the Lanterne Rouge, the unofficial prize for coming last in the race. He and teammate Brian Robinson were the first two British riders ever to finish the Tour.

consumed. They work for a period of time and can genuinely help people lose weight, but by and large, they don't offer long-term solutions and most people end up putting the weight back on pretty quickly.

Still, as they're not endangering health, I'm not going to carp on about them too much! Unless, that is, you're serious about your cycling performance, because none of these diets are devised with an endurance athlete in mind. They lack the abundant carbs, protein, fat and nutrients required and have no flexibility in terms of the demands and schedules of serious training and competition.

Low-carbohydrate diets

Considering carbohydrates make up over half of your calorie intake, it's clear that any attempt to create a calorie deficit will require a reduction in carbs. Now you do the maths: on a ride you will need a minimum of 400 calories an hour, perhaps even double that, and there is a limit to how many calories your body can store – burn over 2000 and you're going to need to replenish or face the dreaded bonk. We have all been there: your vision narrows, you get the shakes and feel like you cannot turn another pedal stroke if your life depends on it. It is not pleasant or pretty and has had many a cyclist heading to the nearest petrol station for a Mars bar and a Coke. As a cyclist, you may be able to lose weight by reducing your carb intake on a limited scale while still maintaining performance levels, or you could cut back on your carbs in the off-season or during injury recovery periods, but leave the

extreme measures to those less obsessed with Lycra and two wheels.

Exclusion diets

There's nothing wrong with having the odd drink – we all need a vice – but if you're going to exclude anything from your diet, make it nutrient-bare alcohol. Denying yourself anything a caveman wouldn't have eaten – cooked dishes, 'acidic' foods, or any substance that is generally prevalent in a normal diet – is limiting your ability to consume a wide variety of nutrients and to actually enjoy your food. When you're managing your weight, it's still important to include all food groups – just adjust the amounts based on your training load.

Meal replacement shakes

When mixed with water, these powders can provide a blend of macronutrients and amino acids that is the equivalent of a meal. They might have their uses as a quick fix when you're pushed for time or too knackered to cook, but as a regular part of your diet not only are they insufficient for the volume of calories and protein you might require, they are also no substitute for the texture, nutrients and experience of real food.

Low-calorie ready meals

I don't wish to speak out of turn, but as a rule, I wouldn't feed these to my dogs! Often tasteless and uninspiring, low-calorie ready meals may be low in calories, fat, salt and sugar, but they can be also be seriously lacking in other nutrients and contain additives.

Vegetarian/vegan

I totally understand that many cyclists are committed to diets that exclude meat and dairy. Personally, however, if you're looking to lose weight and compete as an elite cyclist, I don't recommend that you exclude foods such as meat, fish or eggs from your daily diet. My view is that there is currently no solid, well-researched and credible evidence to prove that a plant-based diet makes you a better athlete. If there was, the cycling governing bodies would be banging the vegan drum – but they're not. I know it's a highly emotive subject, but take time-trialling, where the minute details matter and every split-second counts. The 2019 World Time Trial champions, Rohan Dennis and Chloe Dygert-Owen, both eat a balanced and varied diet that includes meat. If there were performance gains to be had from being vegetarian, perhaps they would consider excluding meat. However, having said that, eating excess amounts of any foodstuff, including meat, is to be avoided, while consuming more fruit and vegetables is only a good thing.

When you're managing your weight, it's still important to include all food groups…

Gluten-free

I personally feel better if I avoid gluten whenever possible. A simple way of working out whether you have an intolerance to gluten is to take it out of your diet for 14 days and see how you feel. Then re-introduce it and see whether you feel better or worse. Just one caveat: give the off-the-shelf, gluten-free products a wide berth. Highly processed products are full of crap, however they are dressed up!

A cyclist can still lose weight without making drastic changes to their diet or lifestyle, but by making some slight alterations you can reduce your calorie intake without affecting your training schedule. The following are some ideas on how this can be achieved.

Exercise portion control

Work out how big your portion sizes need to be to suit your weight-loss programme and stick to them. If you don't have kitchen scales, buy some. And if you do, use them. If you prepare too much food, it's much more likely that you'll eat too much.

Not every day is carb day

Many riders overestimate the amount of carbs they need for a ride. You may well not need as many as you think and if it's a rest or a light training day, you can really cut down.

Be GI-savvy

GI (Glycaemic Index) is a measure of how quickly a food is converted to glucose in the bloodstream. Wholegrain foods, oats, fruit, vegetables, beans and lentils are all low-GI and will provide a slow release of energy, stopping you from having to reach for those sugary snacks too early in the ride.

Save sugar for the ride

Energy bars, cakes and sugary drinks provide an important hit when energy levels are low on the bike. Drip-feeding is key, so it's a case of a little and often – don't wait to start topping up the tank, especially during an intense ride or race.

Protein is the cyclist's friend

Protein – chicken, fish, eggs, etc. – can often be the tastiest part of a meal. Savour and use it, as it provides many benefits, including dulling

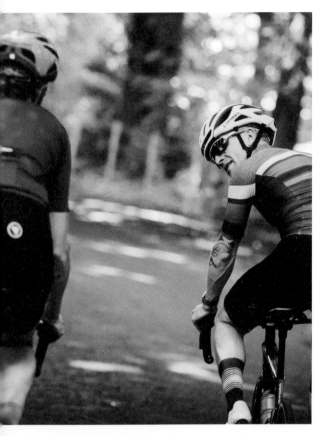

You don't need to fill up on carbs when you're only heading out on an easy ride. Use your light training days to cut down on your calorie intake.

the appetite by slowing the rate of energy release. On rest or light training days include a decent amount of protein (up to 20 grams) in every meal, as it will aid recovery and reduce calories.

Go veg crazy

Low in calories per volume, vitamin- and mineral-rich, metabolism-boosting – vegetables are a godsend. Filling your plate with a combination of cooked and raw vegetables will supercharge your diet. Kale, spinach, broccoli, beetroot, carrots, peppers, cauliflower and green beans are among the veggie kings, but you can't go wrong by shopping in the vegetable aisle.

Love your food

Back to rule number one! I just want to finish this section by saying a little about supplements. There is undoubtedly huge debate about their benefits, but at certain times they might help your body deal with stress, travel, increased training load and/or intensity, or sub-optimal diet. High-strength Omega 3, vitamin D, probiotic and multivitamin supplements are good for general health, and in winter I take vitamin C and zinc to ward off colds. Iron supplements should also be a consideration for female athletes. However, first and foremost, anyone pinning a number on their back needs to make sure that any product they ingest is free of substances prohibited by the World Anti-Doping Agency (WADA). In the UK, look for the Informed Sport logo or similar as a guide. Over-the-counter supplements could be contaminated with banned substances, so if you're going to be competing at any level, avoid them – and that definitely includes any supplements marketed as being able to boost weight loss.

Responsibility for the supplements you put in your body lies solely with you, the individual. Your diet is also down to you. Work out a balanced plan that allows you to achieve your goals and be prepared to fine-tune as necessary, depending on your training and racing schedule, but don't forget that you won't stick to it if you don't enjoy it. Which brings me back yet again to rule number one…

Filling your plate with a combination of cooked and raw vegetables will supercharge your diet.

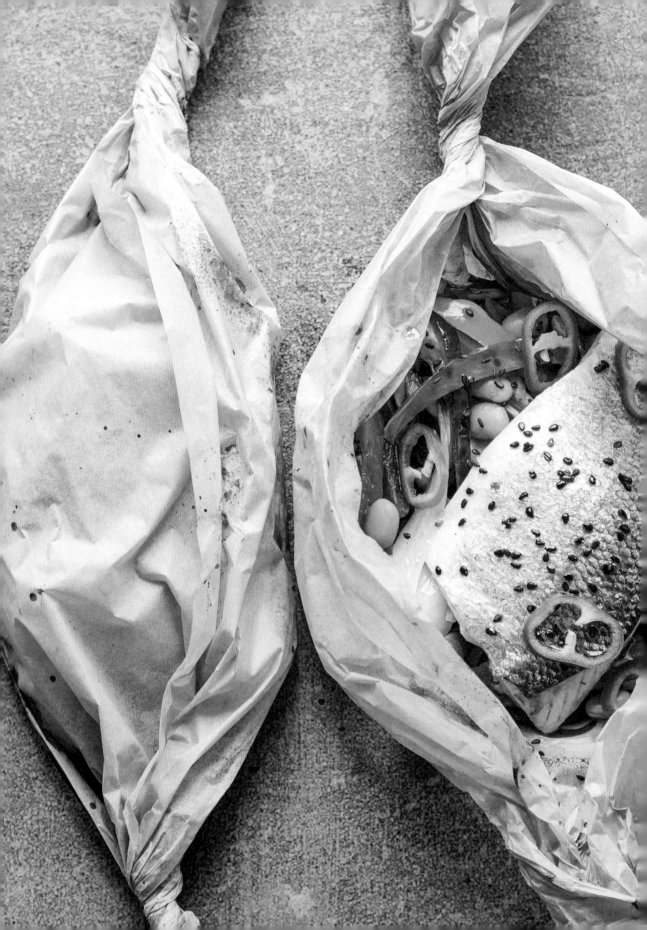

Soft-pedalling days: Lower on energy, still high on taste

If you want to become a better cyclist, learn to cook. That's the advice I always give and on soft-pedalling days there's definitely no excuse for not cooking from scratch, is there? The recipes in this section are ideal for days when your training load is lower and although they may be lower on energy, they are still flavourful. Here, you'll find some tasty soups, including my Murch minestrone (*see* p. 84), a nice Roasted butternut squash and beetroot salad (*see* p. 77), or why not give DIY muesli (*see* p. 78) a go? Days like these are also a good opportunity to experiment a bit with what your body thrives on and what it merely tolerates.

Matcha oat breakfast smoothie

Big old breakfast flavours in a glass! Nice and filling to set you up for a solid day on the bike without feeling 'heavy'.

Serves 2

500 ml (2 cups) unsweetened almond milk

75 g (3 oz) granola

75 g (3 oz) frozen raspberries

2 teaspoons matcha

30 g (1¼ oz) honey

1 ripe banana

1 teaspoon chia seeds

handful of ice cubes

Nutrition per serving:
Energy: 363 kcal
Total carbohydrate: 43 g (of which sugars: 26 g)
Fat: 15 g (of which saturates: 3.4 g)
Fibre: 9.1 g | Protein: 8.7 g | Salt: 0.34 g

LOW-KCAL | MEDIUM-CARB | LOW-PROTEIN

1. Blend all the ingredients together and drink straight away – the smoothie won't sit well in the fridge!

Roasted butternut squash and beetroot salad

A vegetable salad… quite often not the most inspiring of ideas. However, by roasting off the squash and adding some spice and acidity, the humblest of vegetables can be elevated to the next level. Here we use squash, although any root veg you fancy – pumpkin, sweet potato, carrot, parsnip, celeriac – would work well. For a more carb-based meal, add 300 g (11 oz) diced sweet potato to the squash mix. This dish is best served at room temperature.

Serves 2

250 g (9 oz) butternut squash, peeled and diced

100 g (3½ oz) carrots, peeled and diced

1 small red onion, peeled and diced

1 tablespoon olive oil

1 teaspoon sherry vinegar

1 teaspoon BBQ spices

1 teaspoon maple syrup

150 g (5 oz) cooked beetroot

sea salt and freshly ground black pepper

1 large avocado, peeled, pitted and diced

1 teaspoon extra virgin olive oil

squeeze of lemon juice

1 tablespoon toasted pine nuts

good-sized bag of mixed salad leaves to serve

1. Preheat the oven to 150°C/300°F/Gas 2. Meanwhile, in a bowl, mix together the diced squash, carrots and onion with the olive oil, vinegar, BBQ spices and maple syrup. Arrange on a non-stick baking tray and bake in the centre of the oven for 25 minutes.

2. Add the cooked beetroot, stir to combine and cook for a further 5 minutes. When cooked, season well and allow to cool.

3. In a bowl, toss the diced avocado with extra virgin olive oil and lemon juice. Carefully combine with the roasted vegetables and top with pine nuts.

4. Serve with a copious amount of salad leaves.

Nutrition per serving:
Energy: 399 kcal
Total carbohydrate: 29 g (of which sugars: 21 g)
Fat: 26 g (of which saturates: 4.4 g)
Fibre: 9.5 g | Protein: 6.3 g | Salt: 0.27 g

LOW-KCAL | LOW-CARB | LOW-PROTEIN

DIY muesli

Now making your own muesli is so incredibly simple, I have no idea why anyone would actually buy it. The flavour profiles here are my personal favourite… well, this week anyway. Have a play yourself but keep in mind the ratio of oats to dried fruit.

Makes 15 servings (76 g/2.6 oz)

500 g (1 lb 2 oz) rolled oats

100 g (3½ oz) golden raisins

100 g (3½ oz) dried banana (the crispy, sugary stuff), broken into chunks

75 g (3 oz) dried mango, diced

75 g (3 oz) dried apricot, diced

75 g (3 oz) flaked coconut

50 g (2 oz) goji berries

50 g (2 oz) sunflower seeds

50 g (2 oz) pumpkin seeds

50 g (2 oz) flax seeds

4 teaspoons ground cinnamon

Nutrition per serving:
Energy: 321 kcal
Total carbohydrate: 40 g (of which sugars: 14 g)
Fat: 13 g (of which saturates: 5.5 g)
Fibre: 8 g | Protein: 7.7 g | Salt: 0.04 g

LOW-KCAL | MEDIUM-CARB | LOW-PROTEIN

1. Mix all the ingredients together and store in an airtight box – simples! Keeps for 4–6 weeks at room temperature.

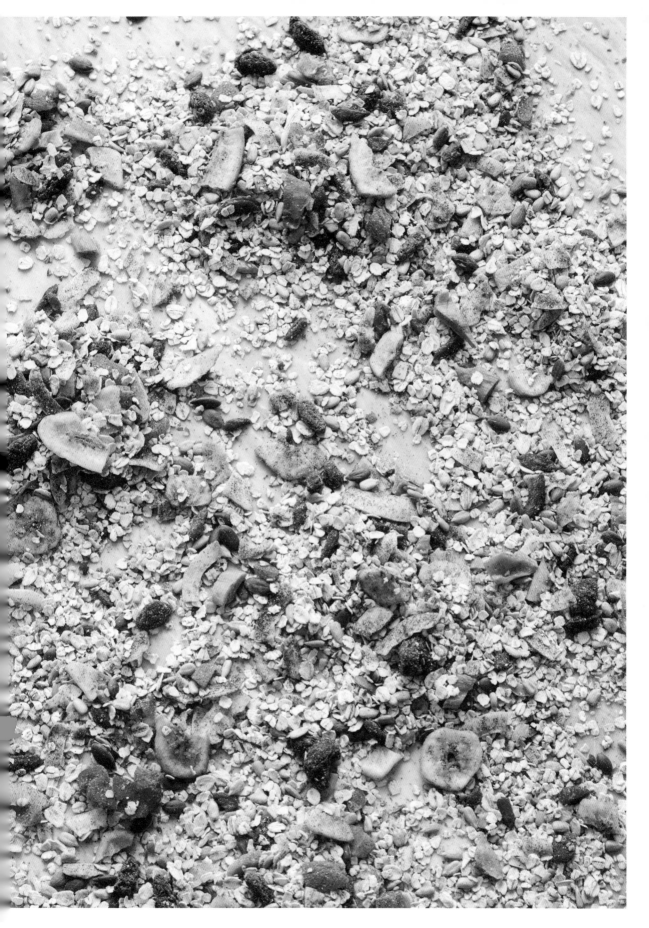

Chillin'

Take your basic 'stretch' mince base (Lentil and beef Bolognese, *see* p. 159) and spice up your life! If you can visit an Asian supermarket locally, you will find there's an array of great-value chilli products that work just as well as fresh chillies (which, being honest, are always a bit hard to judge).

Serves 2

1 teaspoon olive oil

1 teaspoon chopped garlic

1 teaspoon deseeded, chopped red chilli

1 red pepper, deseeded and diced

1 tablespoon tomato purée

1 tin (400 g/14 oz pre-drained weight) kidney beans

300 g (11 oz) stretch mince

cooked rice (75 g/3 oz dry-weight per person) or baked potatoes to serve

Nutrition per serving (without rice/potato):
Energy: 390 kcal
Total carbohydrate: 44 g (of which sugars: 13 g)
Fat: 6.4 g (of which saturates: 1.8 g)
Fibre: 16 g | Protein: 30 g | Salt: 1 g

LOW-KCAL | MEDIUM-CARB | HIGH-PROTEIN

1. Heat the olive oil in a sauté pan. Add the garlic, chilli and diced pepper. Cook over a low heat for 4–5 minutes.

2. Stir in the tomato purée and cook for a further 2 minutes.

3. Next in are the kidney beans. Stir in and simmer for 3 minutes.

4. Add the mince, heat up and served with cooked rice or a baked potato.

Two-for-one: 'Murch magic' mushroom soup and pasta bake

Cunning plan here… work smarter, not harder! I suggest you make a base soup according to the recipe below and, while you're at it, make yourself a banging pasta bake for the next day. Use a third of the soup mix for a cracking wee pasta bake. For a pasta bake for two, add two portions of the mushroom soup, cook 200 g (7 oz) pasta (dry-weight), 250 g (9 oz) cooked chicken and a head of cooked broccoli. Mix in the soup, transfer to an ovenproof dish, top with 60 g (2½ oz) Gruyère and place in an oven preheated to 180°C/350°F/Gas 4 for 15 minutes – tidy!

Makes 4 portions of soup and 2 portions for the pasta bake base

100 g (3½ oz) butter

1 large onion, peeled and finely chopped

2 tablespoons chopped garlic

450 g (1 lb) mixed mushrooms, sliced (chestnut and button work well)

100 g (3½ oz) plain flour

500 ml (2 cups) semi-skimmed milk

1500 ml (3 pints) chicken or vegetable stock

sea salt and freshly ground black pepper

60 g (2½ oz) low-fat crème fraîche

1 bunch of fresh tarragon, chopped

Nutrition per serving:
Energy: 295 kcal
Total carbohydrate: 26 g (of which sugars: 8.8 g)
Fat: 18 g (of which saturates: 11 g)
Fibre: 2.3 g | Protein: 7.9 g | Salt: 2.3 g

LOW-KCAL | LOW-CARB | LOW-PROTEIN

Nutrition per serving (pasta bake):
Energy: 987 kcal
Total carbohydrate: 97 g (of which sugars: 14 g)
Fat: 33 g (of which saturates: 18 g)
Fibre: 11 g | Protein: 72 g | Salt: 3 g

HIGH-KCAL | HIGH-CARB | HIGH-PROTEIN

1. Melt the butter in a large soup pan. Add the onion and garlic and cook over a low heat for 4–5 minutes.

2. Add the mushrooms and cook over a medium heat for a further 5 minutes until slightly coloured.

3. Stir in the flour and cook over a low heat for 3–4 minutes, stirring to make sure the mixture doesn't burn. Gradually add the milk, stirring to ensure no lumps, and then add the stock.

4. Simmer over a low heat for 15–20 minutes, making sure the bottom of the pan does not catch (the mix of 50:50 butter and flour for the 'roux' base is an old-school technique).

5. Allow to cool for 15 minutes and then liquidise and adjust the seasoning.

6. When you come to serving the soup, warm in the pan and then spoon into bowls. Add a dollop of crème fraîche and some chopped tarragon to each one.

Sweet potato tortilla, Vittoria-style

This is a version of a classic Spanish tortilla that I was shown how to make in a local restaurant in the Basque region of Northern Spain while visiting my buddy Pat. My technique uses significantly less oil than the classic method. I also use sweet potato, which I find takes this humble egg dish to another level. The tortilla reheats really well and it's ace to have in the fridge for post-hard ride inhalation!

Makes 4 portions

500 g (1 lb 2 oz) sweet potato (peeled weight)

2 teaspoons BBQ spices

1½ tablespoons olive oil

sea salt and freshly ground black pepper

8 large, free-range eggs

green salad to serve

Nutrition per serving:
Energy: 336 kcal
Total carbohydrate: 27 g (of which sugars: 8.4 g)
Fat: 16 g (of which saturates: 3.9 g)
Fibre: 5.6 g | Protein: 18 g | Salt: 0.77 g

LOW-KCAL | LOW-CARB | MEDIUM-PROTEIN

1. Preheat the oven to 180°C/350°F/Gas 4. Meanwhile, chop the sweet potato evenly and mix in a bowl with the BBQ spices and olive oil. Season well and arrange in a 25 cm (10 in) non-stick ovenproof pan.

2. Place the pan in the centre of the oven and bake for 20–25 minutes until the potato is cooked.

3. While the potato is cooking, whisk up the eggs in a large bowl.

4. OK, for the next stage you need to move fairly quickly as the potato needs to be hot. Remove the pan from the oven (keep the oven on) and then transfer the potato to a large bowl with a slotted spoon – remember, the pan handle will be hot!

5. Take a potato masher and crush the potatoes to a rustic mash, then quickly whisk the potato mix into the beaten eggs, ensuring the mixture is well combined.

6. Using the same pan that you cooked the potato in (there should be enough fat left in the pan), place the pan over a medium heat. Pour in the egg mixture and cook for 2 minutes on the stove, pushing the mixture about with a spatula and loosening from the sides of the pan.

7. Place the tortilla in the oven for 8 minutes or until the top of the egg mixture is firm to the touch. Allow to cool for 2 minutes before slicing into wedges and enjoy with a large handful of greens.

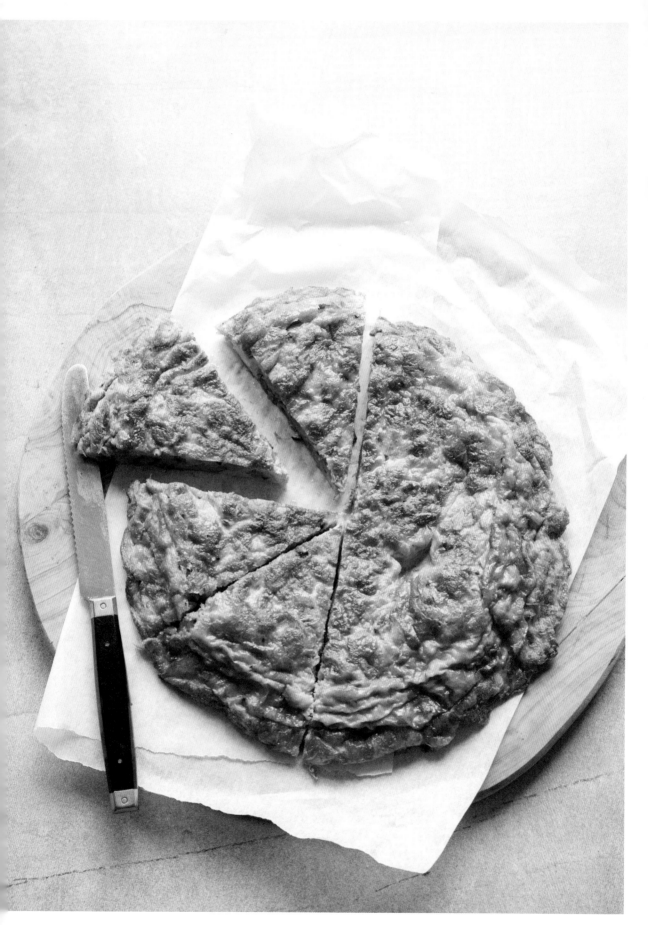

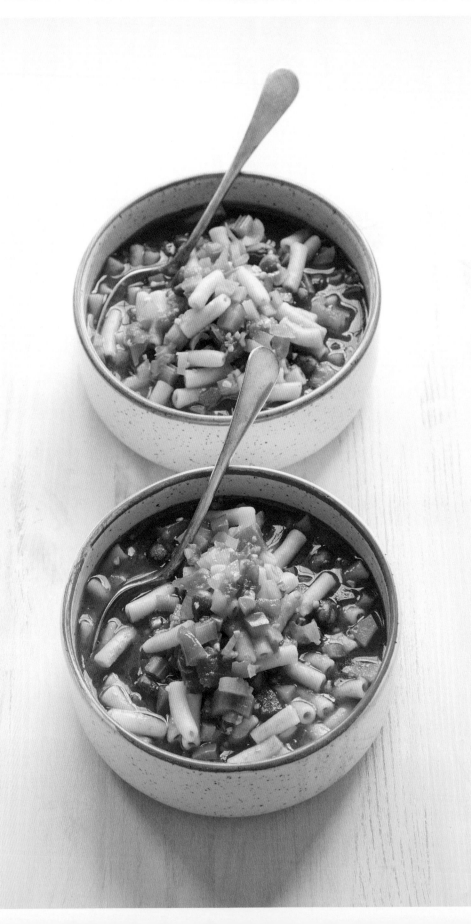

Murch minestrone

Great for a lighter dinner or hearty post-ride lunch! 'Making the minestrone' was one of the very first jobs I was entrusted with on starting out on my culinary journey as a commis chef. Minestrone soup comes from a genre of cuisine referred to as 'Cucina Povera' – literally, 'poor kitchen/poor people's cuisine'. I see this as a way of using humble ingredients and turning them into something special.

When reheating, add a couple of tablespoons of extra stock per portion as the soup will thicken in the fridge.

Makes 6 decent portions

2 tablespoons olive oil

900 g (2 lb) diced mixed veg (celery, onion, carrots, peppers)

2 tablespoons chopped garlic (you can use 'lazy garlic')

1 tin (400 g/14 oz) chopped tomatoes

1500 ml (3 pints) vegetable stock and 500 ml (2 cups) stock for reheating

2 tins cooked beans (borlotti or pinto work best, 400 g/14 oz pre-drained weight)

200 g (7 oz) dry-weight macaroni pasta (you can use gluten-free)

150g (5 oz) fresh diced tomato to finish

1. Heat the olive oil in a large soup pan and fry the veg for 4–5 minutes to release the sweetness.
2. Add the chopped garlic and cook for a further 1–2 minutes.
3. Stir in the tinned tomatoes and stock. Simmer for 15–20 minutes.
4. The next stage is to add the cooked beans and pasta. Simmer for a further 5–8 minutes until the pasta is just cooked (al dente – 'firm to the bite').
5. Stir through the fresh diced tomato at the last minute before transferring to bowls.

Nutrition per serving:
Energy: 323 kcal
Total carbohydrates: 45 g (of which sugars: 13 g)
Fat: 6.1 g (of which saturates: 1 g)
Fibre: 14 g | Protein: 14 g | Salt: 1.6 g

LOW-KCAL | MEDIUM-CARB | MEDIUM-PROTEIN

Smoky green pea broth

A simple light lunch option for days of soft pedalling. Even though this rustic soup is full of flavour, it is surprisingly low in calories. The key here is to roast off the veg to get plenty of flavour in there. Also, the quality of the bacon affects the depth of flavour, so go for nitrate-free if possible. The soup freezes well (allow to cool and transfer to an airtight container, keeps for 4–6 weeks) and it's also cheap to make... no bad news here!

Makes 6 portions

1 tablespoon olive oil

400 g (14 oz) mixed root vegetables (parsnips, carrots, celeriac, onion), peeled and roughly chopped

150 g (5 oz) smoked streaky bacon, roughly chopped

1 teaspoon chopped garlic

250 g (9 oz) dried split green peas

2000 ml (4 pints) chicken stock

sea salt and freshly ground black pepper

Nutrition per serving:
Energy: 175 kcal
Total carboydrate: 13 g (of which sugars: 5.7 g)
Fat: 8.9 g (of which saturates: 2.8 g)
Fibre: 6 g | Protein: 7.8 g | Salt: 2.2 g

LOW-KCAL | LOW-CARB | LOW-PROTEIN

1. Heat the olive oil in a large soup pan. Add the root vegetables and cook over a medium heat for 5–6 minutes until lightly coloured.

2. Add the smoked bacon and garlic. Cook for a further 3 minutes.

3. Stir in the split peas and stock. Bring to the boil and simmer gently for 40–50 minutes until the peas have softened. Stir occasionally so it doesn't catch the bottom of the pan.

4. Allow to cool for 30 minutes, then liquidise. Reheat as many portions as you wish to have and adjust the seasoning.

Jerky butternut squash, sweet potato and carrot soup

Full on flavour, you almost want it to be raining (says no cyclist ever!) when this robust soup is on the go. It freezes really well (allow to cool and transfer to an airtight container, keeps for 4–6 weeks) and would also work really well stirred into cooked pasta and topped with cheese for an easy pasta-type bake.

Serves 6

1 large onion

150 g (5 oz) sweet potatoes

150 g (5 oz) carrots

150 g (5 oz) butternut squash

2 tablespoons olive oil

1 tablespoon jerk seasoning

1 teaspoon smoked paprika

250 g (9 oz) yellow split peas

2500 ml (4½ pints) vegetable stock

sea salt and freshly ground black pepper

small bunch of fresh tarragon

Nutrition per serving:
Energy: 188 kcal
Total carbohydrate: 25 g (of which sugars: 7.5 g)
Fat: 5.9 g (of which saturates: 1.3 g)
Fibre: 5.9 g | Protein: 6.3 g | Salt: 1.5 g

LOW-KCAL | LOW-CARB | LOW-PROTEIN

1. The first job is to trim, peel and roughly dice all the vegetables.

2. Heat the olive oil in a large soup pan, add the vegetables and cook over a medium heat for 5–6 minutes until lightly coloured.

3. Add the jerk seasoning and smoked paprika. Cook for a further 3 minutes.

4. Stir in the yellow split peas and vegetable stock. Bring to the boil and simmer gently for 40–50 minutes until the vegetables and peas have softened. Stir occasionally so it doesn't catch the bottom of the pan.

5. Allow to cool for 30 minutes, then liquidise.

6. Reheat as many portions of soup as you wish to have and adjust the seasoning. Chop the tarragon and sprinkle over the soup just before serving.

Baked ginger and sesame sea bream 'en papillote'

A really lovely way to eat fish, cooking it in its own juices with the amazing flavours of ginger, sesame and soy. It goes without saying that you can use pretty much any fish you fancy for this recipe, but sea bream and cod work particularly well.

Serves 2

2 heads of pak choi, finely sliced

50 g (2 oz) fresh ginger, peeled and finely grated

1 red pepper, deseeded and finely sliced

2 small red onions, peeled and finely sliced

60 g (2½ oz) edamame beans

1 tablespoon sesame oil

2 tablespoons light soy sauce

1 teaspoon sliced and deseeded green chilli

1 teaspoon black sesame seeds

1 teaspoon lime juice

2 x 100 g (3½ oz) sea bream fillets

2 x 35 x 35 cm (14 x 14 in) pieces of greaseproof paper

Nutrition per serving:
Energy: 311 kcal
Total carbohydrate: 21 g (of which sugars: 15 g)
Fat: 12 g (of which saturates: 2.1 g)
Fibre: 4.9 g | Protein: 27 g | Salt: 2.9 g

LOW-KCAL | LOW-CARB | HIGH-PROTEIN

1. Preheat the oven to 200°C/400°F/Gas 6.

2. In a large bowl, combine all the ingredients with the exception of the bream fillets. Stir well.

3. Lay out the greaseproof paper on a worktop.

4. Arrange a quarter of the vegetable mixture in the centre of each paper sheet, then place a fish fillet on top of each one before topping with the remaining vegetables.

5. Draw up the sides of the paper and pour over the cooking juices equally into each parcel before sealing up the sides neatly.

6. Bake in the centre of the oven for 20 minutes then allow to rest for 5 minutes. Transfer to warmed plates, unwrap carefully and enjoy!

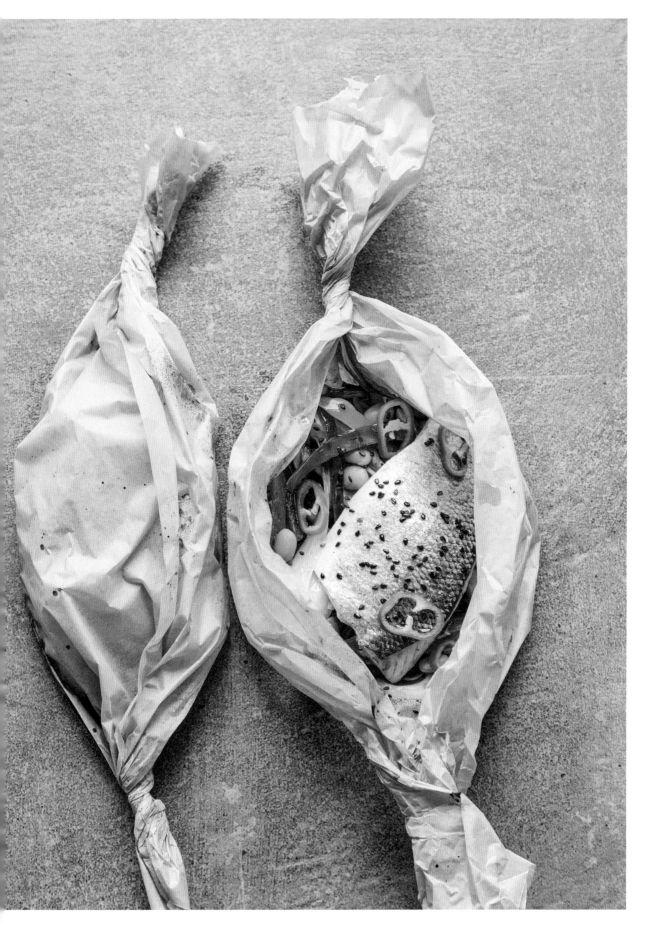

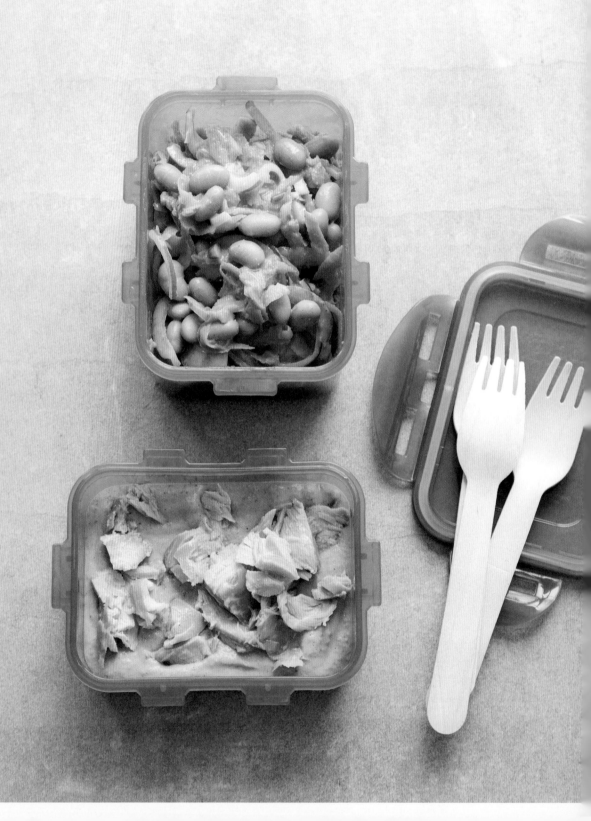

Protein pots

These are a great way of snacking between meals or for pre-ride snack action and way more cost-effective than the shop-bought alternatives. Can be served with sticks of raw veg, crudités-style.

Carrot and edamame protein pots

Edamame beans are one of my fave snacking foods, being high in protein and packed with nutrients with a nutty texture too. I have no idea why they're so expensive in restaurants as they're really cheap when bought from the freezer aisle of the supermarket.

Makes 4 pots – 375 g (13 oz) (snack-size)

300 g (11 oz) carrots, grated

2 small red onions, peeled and finely sliced

100 g (3½ oz) edamame beans

60 g (2½ oz) peanut butter (peanut butter works best but any nut butter will do)

2 teaspoons white wine vinegar

2 tablespoons sweet chilli sauce

4 teaspoons olive oil

sea salt and freshly ground black pepper

bag of mixed salad leaves to serve

Nutrition per serving:
Energy: 282 kcal
Total carbohydrate: 24 g (of which sugars: 20 g)
Fat: 15 g (of which saturates: 2.9 g)
Fibre: 7.4 g | Protein: 9.5 g | Salt: 0.23 g

MEDIUM-KCAL | MEDIUM-CARB | MEDIUM-PROTEIN

1. In a bowl, mix together the grated carrot, onions and edamame beans.
2. In a separate bowl, stir the nut butter, white wine vinegar, sweet chilli sauce and olive oil to form a dressing.
3. Combine the dressing with the salad and adjust the seasoning. Serve with the salad leaves.

Beetroot, feta and chickpea hummus protein pots

A nice change from regular hummus, this recipe also works well with a touch of chilli. It can be kept in the fridge for up to 3 days.

Makes 4 pots – 131 g (4.6 oz) (snack-size)

1 tin cooked chickpeas (400 g/14 oz, 230 g/8 oz drained weight)

150 g (5 oz) pickled cooked beetroot

50 ml (3 tablespoons) olive oil

25 ml (1½ tablespoons) water

pinch of sea salt and freshly ground black pepper

50 g (2 oz) feta, diced

4 teaspoons pumpkin seeds

Nutrition per serving:
Energy: 255 kcal
Total carbohydrate: 11 g (of which sugars: 2.5 g)
Fat: 19 g (of which saturates: 4 g)
Fibre: 3.7 g | Protein: 8 g | Salt: 0.43 g

MEDIUM-KCAL | MEDIUM-CARB | MEDIUM-PROTEIN

1. Strain off the chickpeas and transfer to the bowl of a food processor. Blend with the beetroot, olive oil, water and seasoning to form a smooth paste.

2. Transfer to a bowl, top with diced feta and sprinkle with pumpkin seeds.

Smoked salmon and pea purée protein pots

A classic marriage of salmon and peas, the mint and lemon takes it to the next level. This base would also work well as a larger salad lunch with some cooked new potatoes and a green salad.

Makes 4 pots – 108 g (3.8 oz) (snack-size)

200 g (7 oz) frozen peas, defrosted

70 ml (4 tablespoons) extra virgin olive oil

juice of 1 lemon

a few sprigs of fresh mint

sea salt and freshly ground black pepper

100 g (3½ oz) smoked salmon, finely sliced, to serve

Nutrition per serving:
Energy: 248 kcal
Total carbohydrate: 5.7 g (of which sugars: 3.2 g)
Fat: 20 g (of which saturates: 3.1 g)
Fibre: 2.7 g | Protein: 9.3 g | Salt: 0.54 g

MEDIUM-KCAL | LOW-CARB | MEDIUM-PROTEIN

1. Place the peas in the bowl of a food processor with the olive oil, lemon and mint sprigs. Blend until smooth and season well.

2. Serve with the smoked salmon, either hot or cold.

Avocado, prawn and lemon protein pots

The classic combo of avocado and prawns is almost a throwback to the seventies dinner party. Good fats and protein with minimal preparation required, so no bad news here!

Makes 4 pots – 125 g (4 oz)

1 large avocado, peeled and pitted

200 g (7 oz) peeled prawns

50 g (2 oz) cucumber, finely diced

35 ml (2 tablespoons) extra virgin olive oil

juice of half a lemon

1 teaspoon chia seeds

sea salt and freshly ground black pepper

Nutrition per serving:
Energy: 187 kcal
Total carbohydrate: 1.2 g (of which sugars: 0.7 g)
Fat: 16 g (of which saturates: 2.8 g)
Fibre: 1.8 g | Protein: 8.1 g | Salt: 0 g

MEDIUM-KCAL | LOW-CARB | MEDIUM-PROTEIN

1. Roughly chop the avocado into a bowl and mix with the prawns and cucumber.
2. Stir in the olive oil, lemon juice and chia seeds. Season well and serve.

Poached red fruit with basil and pink peppercorns

When red fruit is in season, this usually means we can't use it fast enough! Gently 'poaching' stretches out the shelf life. The flavour profile also changes when cooked with basil, vinegar and peppercorns, giving the fruit a sweet-and-sour kick. Serve with your morning porridge or pre-bed as a dessert with a generous portion of full-fat Greek yoghurt and a sprinkling of seeds.

With the cooking liquor, once you've removed the fruit you can reduce the mix to a syrup, chill and use as a cordial base with sparkling water.

Serves 6 (snack-size)

800 g (1 lb 7 oz) mixed berries (blueberries, blackberries, strawberries, raspberries)

125 g (4 oz) brown sugar

125 ml (½ cup) water

50 ml (3 tablespoons) sherry vinegar

2 teaspoons dried pink peppercorns

good pinch of freshly ground black pepper

1 teaspoon vanilla extract

1 bunch of fresh basil, chopped

Nutrition per serving:
Energy: 136 kcal
Total carbohydrate: 29 g (of which sugars: 29 g)
Fat: 0.5 g (of which saturates: 0 g)
Fibre: 3.7 g | Protein: 1.3 g | Salt: 0.03 g

MEDIUM-KCAL | MEDIUM-CARB | LOW-PROTEIN

1. Place the berries in a sieve and rinse. Gently pat dry on kitchen paper then transfer to a heatproof bowl.

2. Place the brown sugar and water in a heavy-based pan and set over a medium heat for 10–15 minutes, stirring occasionally, until a light syrup forms.

3. Stir in the sherry vinegar, pink peppercorns and black pepper. Cook for a further 2 minutes before stirring in the vanilla extract.

4. Pour the hot syrup over the berries, stir gently and cover with a clean tea towel. Allow to cool for 1 hour at room temperature, then stir in the basil and place in the fridge overnight to allow the flavours to infuse. The poached fruit can be kept in the fridge for up to 3 days.

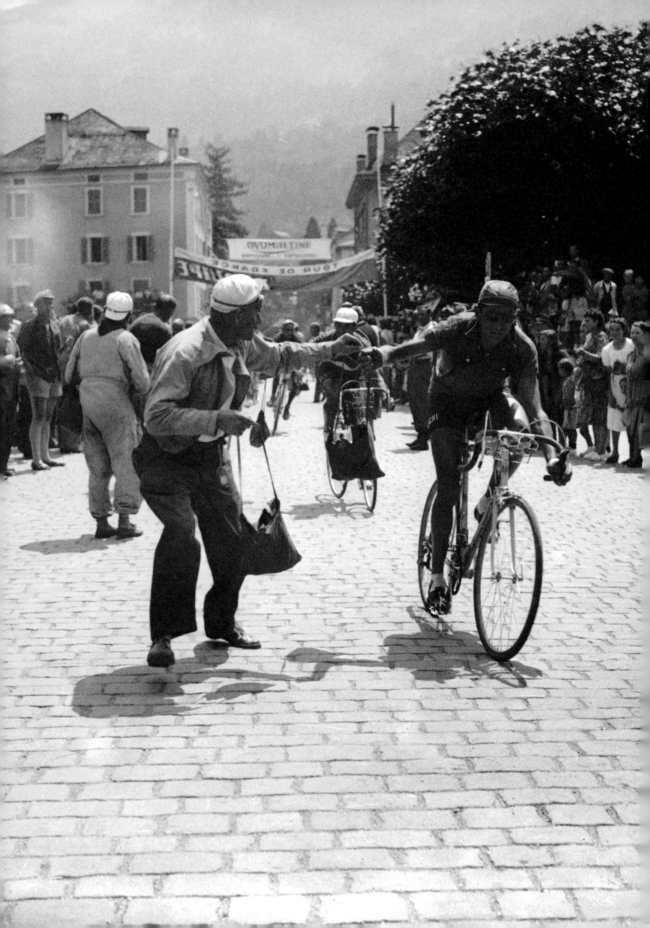

Training for Weight Loss

You're an athlete, right? You might really believe those kilos are going to fly off the minute you pull the Lycra on. Perhaps you think you don't need to watch what you eat, reasoning that when you've added an extra ride to your schedule, it'll burn off that Mars Bar and plenty more besides, and maybe you're right. Maybe you're one of the lucky ones who stay in shape no matter what, but my guess is that you're the same as the rest of us, and if that's true, perhaps you're wondering how come after a month of slogging it out on the road, you've lost nothing but heart.

Legendary Italian cyclist Fausto Coppi during a stage of the 1949 Tour de France. That year Coppi became the first rider to win both the Tour and the Giro d'Italia. He repeated the feat again in 1952.

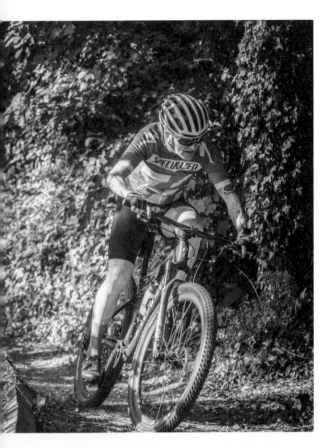

Short periods of riding at full gas can significantly boost fitness. When you only have time for a quick ride on a busy day a high-intensity session can still pay dividends.

The truth is, the 80–20 rule applies as much to athletes as it does to anyone: 80 per cent of any weight loss will be down to modifications in your diet, 20 per cent to changes in your exercise routine. Any extra calorific expenditure on the bike is hard-earned, whereas consumption is easy, and an hour's hard graft in the saddle can be undone by a pastry that takes minutes to eat. Training and diet must go hand in hand, and it's essential you make the most of that 20 per cent.

If you're serious about losing weight, your broad food choices will be related to your goals, so in the off-season, you'll want comforting winter warmers. Pre-season, you'll be looking at lowering your carbs as you focus on getting back on track and, pre-race, pick high-energy, high-carb foods that are easy to digest. On soft-pedalling days, go for foods that are low on energy, but high on taste and on hard days, eat to fuel the machine – which not entirely coincidentally is how the recipes in this book have been categorised!

Make a plan

Many of you reading this book will already have a training schedule and be out on your bikes as much as you need to (or are able to within a normal family and working lifestyle) to train for competition. If the schedule is agreed with your club coaches, then there is little more to be done. To add or change training schedules calculated by an expert who knows you may very well affect performance, so your attention should be focused on how much and when you are eating. However, if your schedule isn't fixed, consider whether you might increase your weekly rides – perhaps extending the route, taking in extra hills or incorporating regular sprints. In this case it may be useful to assess how many calories you're burning on a ride. You can base a rough estimate on an assumption that an 80 kg rider doing an average of in excess of 20 mph for an hour will burn 1000 calories – online calculators can supply figures for other weights and speeds – although this ignores a host of other factors, including the fitness of the rider, the gradient and the presence of head or tail winds, all of which could alter the calculation significantly.

Apps such as Strava (www.strava.com) or Training Peaks (www.trainingpeaks.com) can give a more helpful indication of energy output, but these can still be well wide of the mark unless synced to a heart rate monitor. Where they are useful is in maintaining or improving your efforts from day to day, but it would be unwise to fine-tune your diet according to the results. More useful are power meters, a tool familiar to anyone who has watched or participated in elite cycling. These measure how hard you are pushing on the pedals multiplied by how fast you are pedalling. While cyclists look at the results in watts to reveal the power they are creating, those looking to lose weight may be more interested in the kilojoule figure. There are roughly 4 kJ per food calorie, but only around 25 per cent of energy is transferred to the pedals. So, handily, the body's inefficiency on the bike means the kilojoule figure is equivalent to the number of calories. Power meters have historically been expensive, but are now becoming more affordable with a vast array of options out there. Bob Tobin at Cycle Power Meters is an expert in recommending the appropriate gadget for your budget (www.cyclepowermeters.com).

In the zone

Coaches' and nutritionists' views on training for weight loss have changed over the last couple of decades and continue to be debated. Much of the argument centres on the effectiveness of training in what is termed the 'fat-burning zone'. This zone, when the body sources energy from fat rather than glycogen stored in the muscles and liver, is said to be around 70 per cent of your maximum heart rate (found by subtracting your age from 220).[9] In this zone – a moderate-paced ride – the body may burn 50 per cent of the calories from fat, but the zone exponents claim that at higher intensities the body may only burn 35 per cent from fat, making higher intensities less effective for weight loss.

So far, so clear. However, those debunking the fat-burning zone myth counter that at higher intensities more calories are burned in total and therefore more fat calories overall. What's a poor cyclist to do? Fortunately – or unfortunately – you have no choice. You're going to need to put away some serious hours in the saddle in order to build stamina and muscle endurance, but high intensity interval training (HIIT) has a vital place, too. These short bursts of riding at full gas can significantly boost fitness, are easier to fit into a busy working week and can also aid weight loss. Research by the *British Journal of Sports Medicine* in 2019 found participants in a variety of sports lost 28.5 per cent more weight by performing brief HIIT sessions.[10] Although scientists are

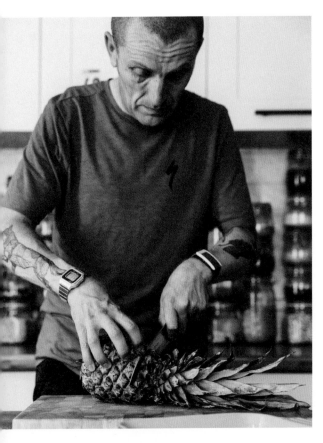

Cooking with fresh ingredients is the last thing you want to do after a hard day on the saddle, so prepare your meals in advance when you have plenty of time.

unclear exactly why this should be the case, some of it is clearly due to longer sessions stimulating appetite and leading to over-refuelling, while some is down to the longer-term effects of HIIT on your metabolism – the rate at which calories are burned by your body.

Metabolic action

Each person has a different resting metabolic rate (RMR) – the number of calories required just to stay alive. The body converts carbohydrates and fat into that energy, and although our RMR is largely predetermined by our genes, it can change. As you get fitter, you will burn more calories as muscles constantly use energy whereas fat uses none. There can also be some increase in metabolic rate for the 12 hours following strenuous exercise as the body deals with muscle damage and makes other repairs. We can train our metabolism to seek the bulk of energy from carbs or from fat as well. Although for weight loss it's ideal to convert more fat, we need to be careful to preserve the carbohydrate metabolic pathways for those long rides and we can do this by fine-tuning our diet and training.

For some people, fasted training – cycling on as few carbs as possible – can help the body look to fat for energy. For health reasons, I wouldn't advise anyone to take this to extremes, but a pre-breakfast, 90-minute ride (taking advantage of the fact that you've been 'fasting' while you were asleep) should be fine for most people. The theory says that with limited carbs available, the body will turn to fat for its energy and this is backed up by some scientific research and plenty of anecdotal evidence.[11] Some caveats though: keep your riding to low- or moderate intensity; if you struggle, sip on a protein drink or, before your next attempt, try a protein-only breakfast prior to the ride; and always remember to have your normal breakfast after the ride in order to restore depleted muscle glycogen.

Incorporating low-carb days into your diet plan can also help your metabolism tip towards burning fat – have a look at the recipes in the Pre-season section (*see* pp. 50-67) for some ideas. On rest or low-intensity days, try transferring to a diet with a high protein ratio. Only around 25 per cent of your daily calories should come from carbohydrate and these should be consumed before and after the ride, with other meals consisting of as few carbs as possible.

Riding in the fat-burning zone, interval training, fasted training and low-carb days can all help a weight-loss programme, but this will all be in vain if you don't control what you're eating. You will never be able to ride yourself thin, but you can use apps such as Strava, MyFitnessPal or similar to keep a daily log of everything you eat, what kind of training you've done and your body fat or weight, because these will help you streamline your riding and eating for maximum effect. Personally, I only have to look at food to put on weight and if you're one of those 'lucky ones' – or annoying gits – I mentioned earlier, then I'm pleased for you, honestly I am! For the rest of us, as the great three-time winner of the Tour de France Greg LeMond reputedly said, 'It never gets easier, you just go faster,' but eat and train the right way and I guarantee you'll drop those kilos. And, as I'm fairly sure LeMond never said, remember, sweat is really just fat crying.

I only have to look at food to put on weight and if you're one of those 'lucky ones' I'm pleased for you, honestly I am!

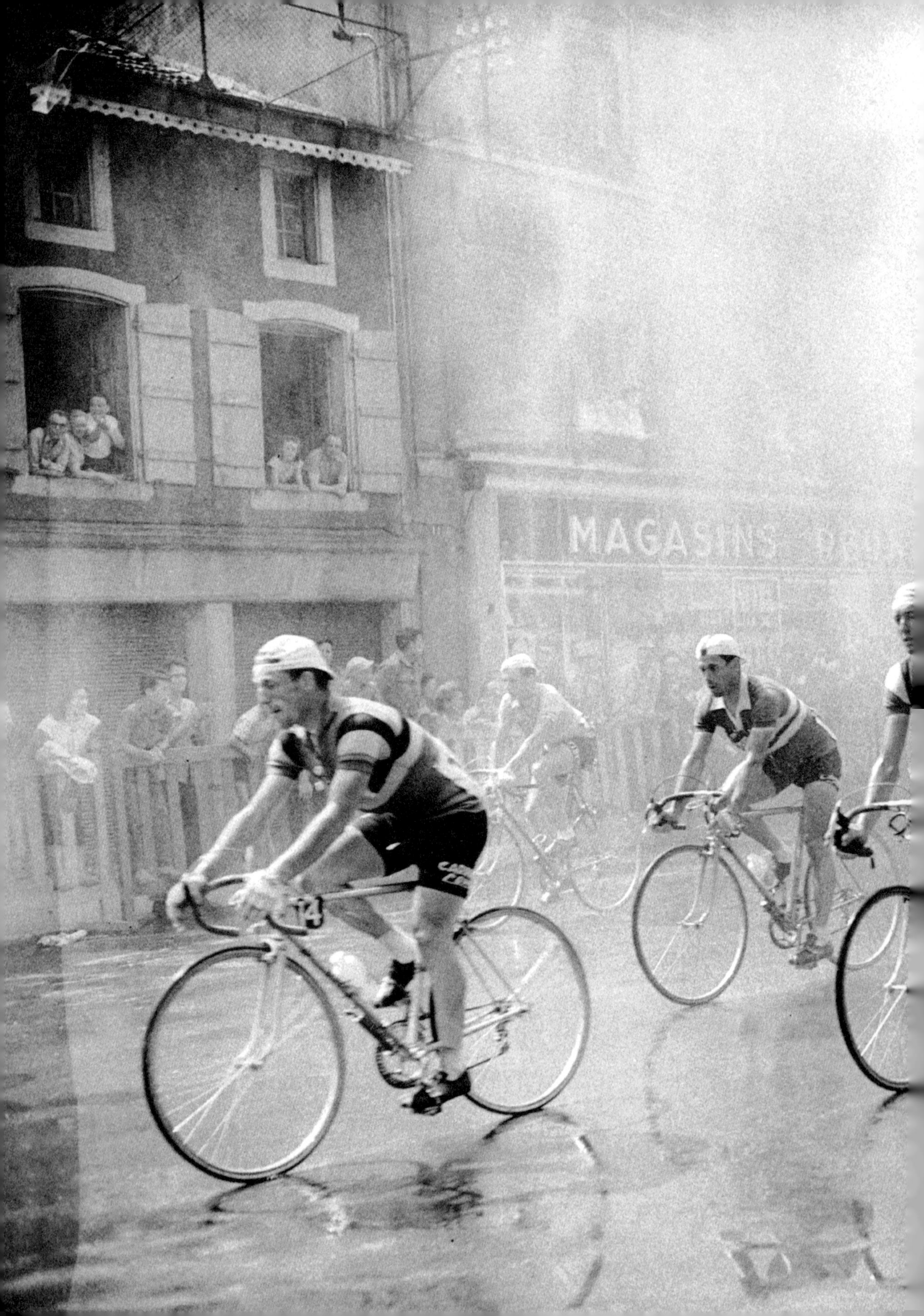
MAGASINS
14

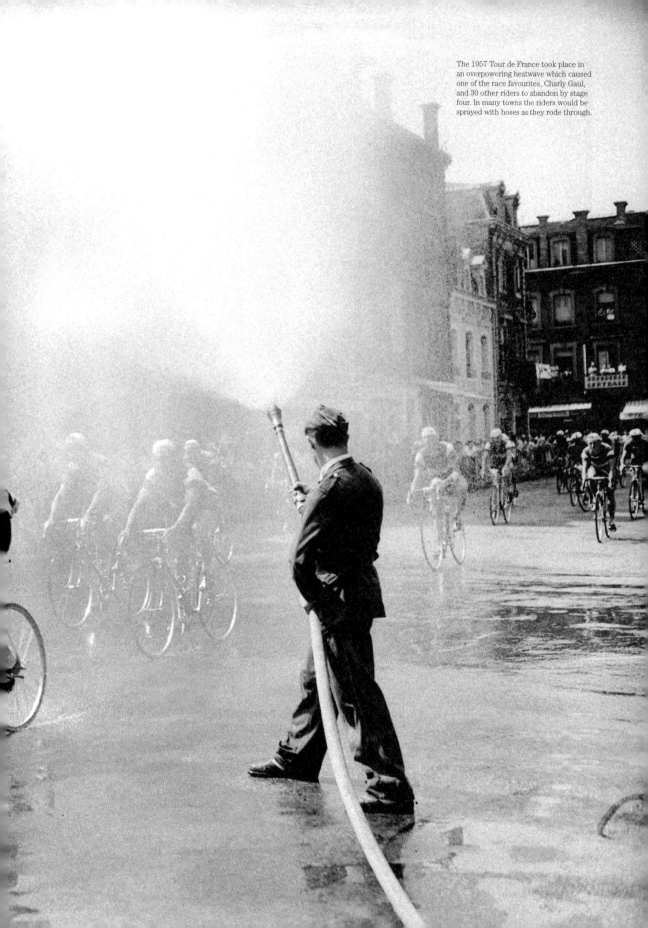

The 1957 Tour de France took place in an overpowering heatwave which caused one of the race favourites, Charly Gaul, and 30 other riders to abandon by stage four. In many towns the riders would be sprayed with hoses as they rode through.

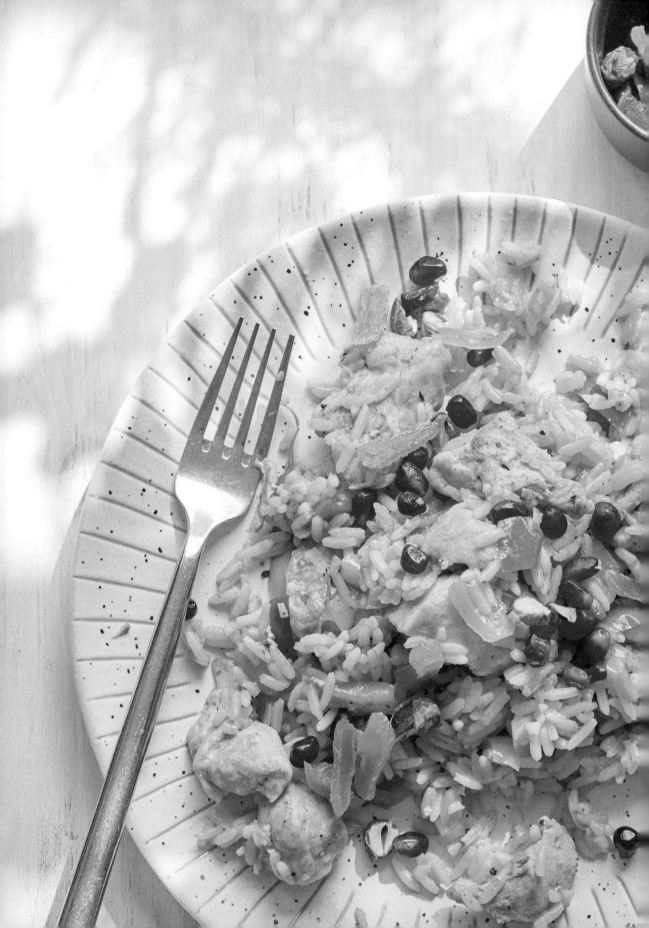

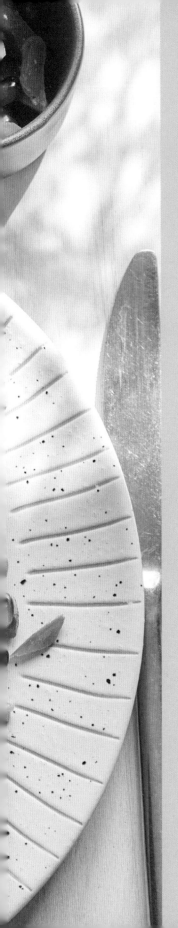

Pre-race: Easy-to-digest, high-energy and high-carb

In terms of what you eat pre-race – and that means the preceding day as well as the race day itself – it needs to be high-carb and easy to digest. The latter is crucial, because the last thing you want as you swing into the saddle is to feel bloated and uncomfortable. Have your protein the night before and get a good night's sleep to aid digestion. Don't skip breakfast, either – even if you're nervous and it's the last thing you feel like – and make it heavy on the carbs, because they will deliver the energy to get you through. Oh, and make sure you're fully hydrated, too.

Pumpkin-spiced bircher muesli

This is a nice way to incorporate veggies into breakfast. It can also be used as a post-training pick-me-up. The humble pumpkin is hugely versatile. My mate Tim and his family farm the most premium of pumpkins, 'Crown Prince', meaning we have a regular supply when they are in season.

If pumpkins are not available, butternut squash or carrot work pretty well too. You can also use regular apple juice instead of apple and mango.

Makes 2 portions

200 g (7 oz) grated pumpkin

2 teaspoons cinnamon

pinch of allspice

2 teaspoons chia seeds

100 g (3½ oz) low-fat Greek yoghurt

100 g (3½ oz) rolled oats

250 ml (1 cup) apple and mango juice

1 tablespoon maple syrup

Nutrition per serving:
Energy: 347 kcal
Total carbohydrate: 57 g (of which sugars: 23 g)
Fat: 5.5 g (of which saturates: 0.9 g)
Fibre: 8.2 g | Protein: 13 g | Salt: 0.18 g

LOW-KCAL | MEDIUM-CARB | MEDIUM-PROTEIN

1. Mix all the ingredients together in a large bowl, stirring well. Cover and place in the fridge overnight, then enjoy!

Sweet and spicy chilli salmon

This is a cracking meal for a hard day, being high in carbs and calories. In fact, it's quite unusual as you normally associate lots of calories with being full/feeling bloated – ideal then if you are pumped full of sports nutrition product and still need to top up. Also, it would be normal to think that fish with rice and veg is low-calorie… in this case it's not!

Serves 2

2 x 150 g (5 oz) salmon fillets

Marinade

100 g (3½ oz) sweet chilli sauce

2 teaspoons Thai fish sauce

2 teaspoons light soy sauce

2 teaspoons olive oil

freshly ground black pepper

Stir-fry rice

1 tablespoon olive oil for frying

1 onion, peeled and finely diced

150 g (5 oz) chopped mixed greens (mangetout, green peppers, green beans)

300 g (11 oz) pre-cooked rice

150 g (5 oz) defrosted frozen peas

small bunch of fresh coriander, chopped

2 tablespoons light soy sauce

1 teaspoon fennel seeds

1 teaspoon sesame seeds

1. Preheat the oven to 190°C/375°F/Gas 5. Meanwhile, mix together all the ingredients for the marinade in a bowl. Place the salmon in an ovenproof dish and pour over the marinade, ensuring the salmon is well-coated.

2. Place the salmon in the centre of oven and bake uncovered for 15–20 minutes until cooked through.

3. Once the salmon has been baking for 10 minutes, heat some olive oil in a frying pan. Gently fry the onion in the oil for 2–3 minutes over a medium heat.

4. Add the chopped mixed greens to the pan and cook for a further 2 minutes. Now add the rice and peas, turn up the heat and cook over a high heat for 3–4 minutes, stirring. At the last minute, stir in the coriander and soy sauce.

5. Finish off the salmon by sprinkling over the fennel and sesame seeds. Pour the cooking juices from the salmon over the rice and serve.

Nutrition per serving:
Energy: 923 kcal
Total carbohydrate: 97 g (of which sugars: 42 g)
Fat: 37 g (of which saturates: 6.3 g)
Fibre: 10 g | Protein: 45 g | Salt: 4.4 g

HIGH-KCAL | HIGH-CARB | HIGH-PROTEIN

Cheryl's coconut oat balls

An easy-to-make wee snack to have on the bike! This recipe is one I have 'borrowed' from my friend Cheryl, one of the soigneurs at British Cycling. I watched her many times when she threw a lot of ingredients in a bowl and this magical little tasty energy ball came out at the end. Now I'm not one for winging it so I devised a cunning plan to do an actual recipe that works and could be repeated without having Cheryl look over my shoulder! Most of us don't have the skills to just throw stuff together.

Makes 15 x 40 g (1½ oz) energy balls (snack-size)

200 g (7 oz) gluten-free oats

150 g (5 oz) pitted dates

100 g (3½ oz) runny honey

100 g (3½ oz) coconut and peanut butter (any nut butter is fine)

3 teaspoons chia seeds

3 teaspoons desiccated coconut

pinch sea salt flakes

1. In the bowl of a food processor, blend the oats, dates, honey and nut butter to form a coarse paste.

2. Add the chia seeds, coconut and sea salt, and blend until the mixture comes together.

3. Remove from the blender and on a work surface roll into balls with your hands. Refrigerate for up to 7 days in an airtight box.

Nutrition per serving:
Energy: 158 kcal
Total carbohydrate: 22 g (of which sugars: 12 g)
Fat: 5.4 g (of which saturates: 2.2 g)
Fibre: 2.9 g | Protein: 3.5 g | Salt: 0.1 g

MEDIUM-KCAL | MEDIUM-CARB | LOW-PROTEIN

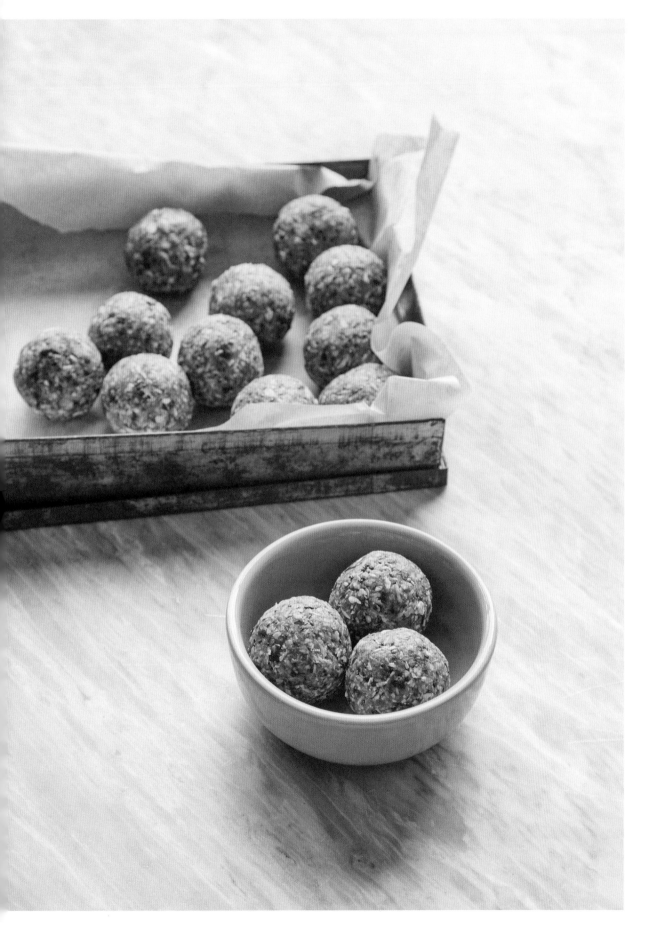

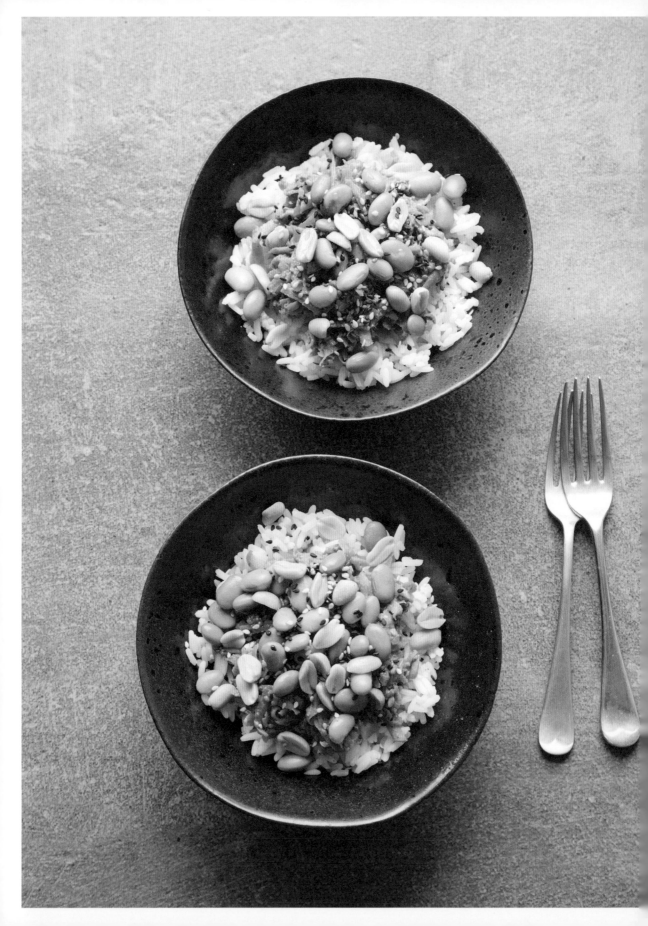

Nutty carrot slaw with edamame beans

Necessity is the mother of invention… I literally made this recipe up at a track World Cup as I needed an extra salad-type meal and had run out of food! True story. It went down so well with the riders that I wrote up the recipe. Here the humble carrot is turned into something a bit special with the addition of some spice and nut butter. Edamame beans take care of protein levels. If the carnivore in you longs for some meat, some Teriyaki chicken (*see* p. 138) works so well with this dish.

Serves 2, plus cheeky little portion leftover for lunch

100 g (3½ oz) edamame beans (usually found near the frozen peas in supermarkets)

75 g (3 oz) white rice (dry-weight per person)

sea salt and freshly ground black pepper

2 tablespoons salted peanuts to serve

1 teaspoon sesame seeds to serve

Slaw

90 g (3½ oz) peanut butter

4 teaspoons white wine vinegar

60 g (2½ oz) sweet chilli sauce

35 g (1½ oz) soy sauce

30 g (1¼ oz) chia seeds

380 g (13¼ oz) grated carrot

1. Make a smooth paste by mixing together the peanut butter, white wine vinegar, sweet chilli sauce, soy sauce and chia seeds in a large bowl.

2. Combine the dressing with the grated carrot to make a slaw and refrigerate for 15–20 minutes.

3. Cook the edamame beans and rice according to the directions on the packs. Season and set aside.

4. Keep it simple: have a bowl of rice and top with the edamame beans and a generous portion of slaw. Served topped with salted peanuts and sesame seeds.

Nutrition per serving:
Energy: 795 kcal
Total carbohydrate: 89 g (of which sugars: 24 g)
Fat: 33 g (of which saturates: 6.5 g)
Fibre: 16 g | Protein: 29 g | Salt: 2.6 g

HIGH-KCAL | HIGH-CARB | HIGH-PROTEIN

Risotto-ish with red lentils

Medium hard day's training fodder, this take on a risotto has a lovely texture and flavour profile, and is a complete meal in one pan. It's also suitable for our vegan friends.

Makes 2 portions

2 tablespoons olive oil

1 small onion, peeled and diced

200 g (7 oz) carrots, trimmed, peeled and diced

1 large red pepper, deseeded and diced

100 g (3½ oz) sweet potatoes, peeled and diced

130 g (4¼ oz) Arborio (risotto) rice

100 g (3½ oz) red lentils

850 ml (3½ cups) vegetable stock

sea salt and freshly ground black pepper

small bunch of chopped tarragon to serve

Nutrition per serving:
Energy: 691 kcal
Total carbohydrate: 109 g (of which sugars: 18 g)
Fat: 17 g (of which saturates: 3.6 g)
Fibre: 11 g | Protein: 21 g | Salt: 4.2 g

HIGH-KCAL | HIGH-CARB | HIGH-PROTEIN

1. Heat the olive oil in a large sauté pan, add all the vegetables and cook over a medium heat for 2–3 minutes.

2. Add the rice and lentils and stir into the vegetables.

3. Now pour in the stock and bring to the boil. Simmer for 18–20 minutes until the liquid has been absorbed and the lentils have softened.

4. Remove from the heat, adjust the seasoning and allow to rest for 4 minutes. Transfer to warmed plates or bowls and serve sprinkled with tarragon.

Pasta 'Barlow'

The perfect pre-hard ride meal that can be knocked up in 10 minutes. This is a take on a rapid carbonara, which I was shown how to cook by a really quick marathon runner mate. So simple, but so tasty, I often eat it straight from the pan.

Serves 2

1 teaspoon salt

250 g (9 oz) dry-weight spaghetti

1 tablespoon olive oil

200 g (7 oz) smoked back bacon, cut into strips

2 large free-range eggs

sea salt and freshly ground black pepper

50 g (2 oz) Parmesan, grated, plus extra to serve

Nutrition per serving:
Energy: 937 kcal
Total carbohydrate: 86 g (of which sugars: 3.8 g)
Fat: 37 g (of which saturates: 14 g)
Fibre: 5.8 g | Protein: 62 g | Salt: 3.6 g

HIGH-KCAL | HIGH-CARB | HIGH-PROTEIN

1. Bring a large saucepan of water to a rolling boil, add a teaspoon of salt and cook the spaghetti until al dente (firm to the bite) according to the pack directions.

2. When the pasta is halfway there, heat the olive oil in a large saucepan, add the bacon and fry over a medium heat for 4–5 minutes.

3. Whisk the eggs in a small bowl and season well. Be careful not to add too much salt as the bacon will take care of this.

4. When your pasta is al dente, drain well, remove the pan of bacon from the heat and immediately add the cooked pasta with the whisked eggs.

5. Add the grated Parmesan and stir thoroughly to combine. The key here is to get this dish out while the pasta and bacon are still hot so the egg cooks into a creamy sauce. It's best served straight from the pan and topped with extra Parmesan and freshly ground black pepper, if liked.

Old-school chicken, apricot and pomegranate pilaf

This is very much an old-school cooking technique, which I learnt a lifetime ago at college! The recipe is similar nutritionally to a risotto but has a different cooking technique and flavour profile. Long-grain rice can break down if messed about with too much so avoid over-stirring once cooked.

Serves 2 with a portion left for lunch

2 tablespoons olive oil

1 medium onion, deseeded and diced

1 red pepper, deseeded and diced

1 yellow pepper, deseeded and diced

1 tablespoon chopped garlic

1 tablespoon BBQ seasoning

2 teaspoons turmeric

500 g (1 lb 2 oz) chicken breast, diced

250 g (9 oz) long-grain rice

800 ml (3¼ cups) chicken stock (plus extra 200 ml/¾ cup to add during cooking, if required)

12 dried apricots, diced

75 g (3 oz) pomegranate seeds

25 g (1 oz) chopped pistachios

Nutrition per serving:
Energy: 787 kcal
Total carbohydrate: 100 g (of which sugars: 29 g)
Fat: 17 g (of which saturates: 2.9 g)
Fibre: 13 g | Protein: 52 g | Salt: 4 g

HIGH-KCAL | HIGH-CARB | HIGH-PROTEIN

1. Preheat the oven to 190°C/375°F/Gas 5. Add olive oil to a large ovenproof dish, then add the diced onion, peppers, garlic, BBQ seasoning and turmeric. Place in the oven for 5–6 minutes.

2. Remove the dish from the oven, add the chicken and return to the oven for a further 5 minutes.

3. Remove the dish from the oven once more, add the rice and the stock. Cover with foil and return to the oven for 20–25 minutes until the liquid has absorbed and the rice is tender. Check after 15 minutes and add more stock, if necessary.

4. Transfer to warmed plates or bowls and serve topped with apricots, pomegranate seeds and pistachios.

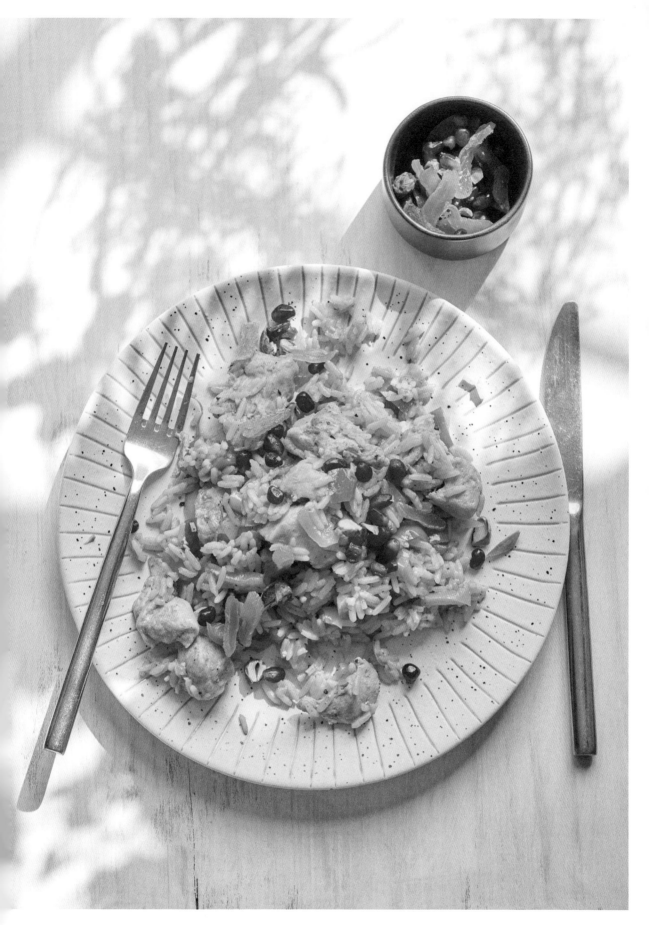

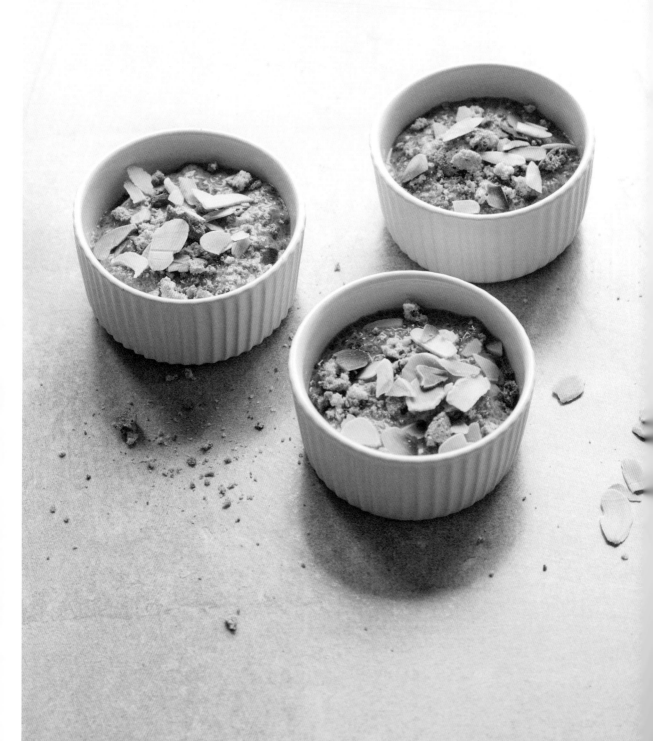

Pre-bed chia puddings with sour cherry and almond

Chef time… With the classic flavour profile of cherry and almond, you can't go wrong. Nerd time… Cherries are one of the few natural food sources of melatonin, the chemical that helps regulate your body clock, so are a great sleep aid. Researchers recommend having concentrated sour cherry juice 60–90 minutes before bed so make this up earlier in the day for a pre-bed snack.

Makes 4 portions (snack-size)

40 g (1½ oz) chia seeds

250 ml (1 cup) unsweetened almond milk

1 tablespoon runny honey

1 tablespoon ground almonds

40 g (1½ oz) cherry concentrate

30 g (1¼ oz) chopped dried cherries

60 g (2½ oz) Amaretti biscuits

1 tablespoon toasted flaked almonds to serve

Nutrition per serving:
Energy: 233 kcal
Total carbohydrate: 29 g (of which sugars: 25 g)
Fat: 9.1 g (of which saturates: 0.8 g)
Fibre: 5.3 g | Protein: 6 g | Salt: 0.1 g

MEDIUM-KCAL | MEDIUM-CARB | LOW-PROTEIN

1. In a small jug, mix together the chia seeds, almond milk, honey, ground almonds and cherry concentrate. Place in the fridge.

2. After 15 minutes, stir the mixture to ensure that it does not settle and separate. Repeat this process a few times over 90 minutes, then leave for 3 hours.

3. To assemble the puddings, spoon the chopped dried cherries into 4 small ramekins. Place the Amaretti biscuits in a small plastic bag, seal and crush with a rolling pin, before adding to the ramekins. Spoon over the cherries.

4. Then divide the chia pudding mix between the ramekins.

5. Refrigerate overnight or make up in the morning before having pre-bed. Sprinkle with toasted almond flakes just before serving.

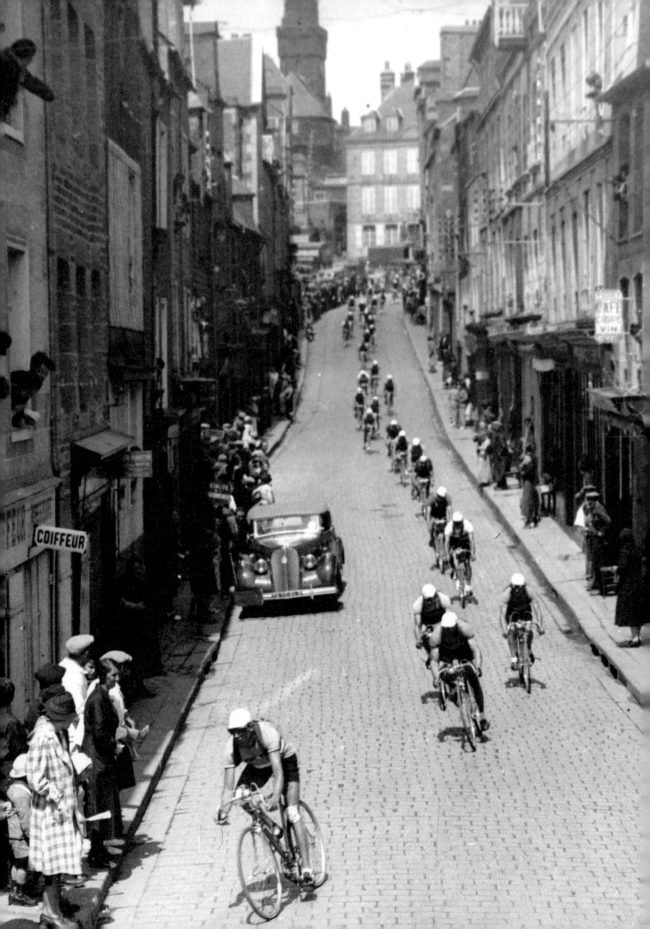

The Fine Line

What's in your musette does matter. Back in
the day they were stuffed with sandwiches
and sugar lumps. In modern times they
usually contain energy bars, gels and a sports
drink, but whether you're lucky enough to
grab one from an outstretched hand at the
side of the road or you've been carrying it
with you since you set off this morning, what's
inside it counts. What you bring with you and
what you leave behind is tricky, though – it's a
fine line and one you're going to have to cycle
along with care.

The race is on as the Tour de France riders
pass through Bressy. In the 1930s riders
entered the Tour in national and French
regional teams. It was a hit with the public,
especially as the French national team won
the first five of these new-style editions.

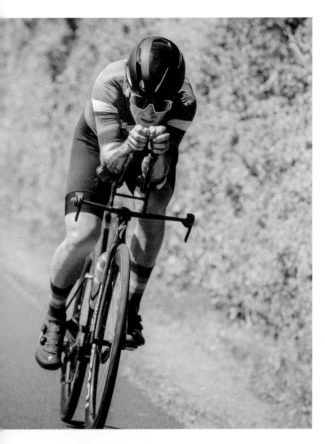

You usually shouldn't need to eat during short time trials, so pre-race nutrition is key to your performance. Eat regularly and healthily throughout the day in preparation for your ride.

In an ideal world, you would take on exactly the right amount of carbs before setting off on a training ride or race and take with you food containing precisely the energy required to complete the ride. Unfortunately, you'll never get it consistently right – an occasional wobble from time to time is to be expected – but experimentation and experience can help get you near the mark.

As discussed earlier, restricting calories (or fasting) before a ride is something that you should consider very carefully and it's certainly inadvisable when embarking on a hard training ride or a race. Similarly, trying to eliminate or cut down your calorie intake during a ride can lead to demotivation, weakness and maybe even bonking. On the other hand, excessive carbo-loading or on-bike refuelling are easy ways to wreck a carefully planned weight-loss programme. The recipes in this book are all calorie-counted and come with a nutritional breakdown, so if you pick one from, say, the Hard days section (*see* pp. 150-177), you know it will deliver the power punch you need.

On the bike

Your body can only store 2000 calories in carbs. That will probably last you for 90 minutes to two hours of solid riding, but once this supply runs down, your body will use its fat reserves for energy. Now that might appeal in terms of losing weight, but it's far from ideal when you're far from home or at a crucial point in the race. This turnover in energy takes place slowly, but it can quickly creep up on you and leave you feeling weak and under-powered. The best option is to pre-empt this by regularly refuelling with bite-sized healthy snacks, such as a banana, some nuts, dried fruit, a homemade oat bar or by taking regular small gulps from an energy drink sachet, because even in events that last less than an hour, a top up of carbs can be beneficial to performance.

So where does this leave the cyclist's 'friend', the energy gel? These gels can be a godsend as they provide carbs in a formula that has been designed to be quickly absorbed into the bloodstream. Most energy gels (and bars) contain around 100 calories and can take effect in 10 to 15 minutes, so they're really useful if you're approaching a tough climb or a final sprint, and can certainly help sustain you over a longer race, but just like any other aspect of your riding, you need to practise using them during training. Try taking them during your race-paced sessions or harder rides so that when you come to take one in a race you know how your body will respond.

Off the bike

When you do dismount, you'll be hungry – probably *very* hungry – but try to avoid reactive eating by planning your training schedule and food plan so that they work together, and the post-ride decisions you make about what to eat aren't dictated by emotion.

After a hard ride you're going to require protein. Your muscles have been working for hours and need some TLC. Again, don't overdo it. Between 10 and 20 grams of protein will be enough for a post-ride refuel. A scoop of whey powder contains 30 grams of protein, but is also over 200 calories. You'll need to replenish some carbs too, but once you're back on two legs – or even lying down – you don't need a chocolate bar, a bag of chips or a bowl of pasta. Instead, reach for a fruit smoothie or maybe a frittata or protein pot.

After a hard ride you're going to require protein. Your muscles have been working for hours and need some TLC.

Constantly thinking or talking about food or frequently missing meals are good indicators that your mindset around food could be better...

You can kickstart your recovery as soon as you're out of the saddle. In fact, ideally, you should eat within 15 minutes of finishing your ride, because the enzyme that stores carbs as glycogen in your muscles is particularly active straight after exercise, so the faster you can consume calories the better – as long as they're the right calories, of course. However, replenishing protein, carbs, fluids and electrolytes also needs to be ongoing for several hours and certainly the first 60–90 minutes after your ride. Within a couple of hours of the ride, eat a fairly substantial meal so your body can continue replacing energy stores and accessing the amino acids and fats that will help repair your muscles. However, there's some evidence to suggest it's better to eat a little and often, so after an intense session some elite athletes consume smaller portions every two hours for six or so hours, especially if they're due to ride again later or the following day.

Remember, though, these strategies are for when you've really pushed yourself and expended a significant amount of energy. After your regular ride to work or an hour or so of steady cycling you will definitely have burned some calories, which is all to the good, but your body should be able to handle that and there is no need to eat immediately – just wait for your next meal as normal and save yourself the calories.

The psychology of eating

Many of us, including elite athletes, have a complicated relationship with food. It is entirely possible to be light, lean, fit – and very unhealthy. I've certainly seen elite athletes with eating disorders and even a very serious condition called relative energy deficiency in sport (RED-S). It's caused by insufficient calorie intake and/or excessive training, resulting in a negative energy balance over time, and can adversely affect not only performance, but also long-term health, including osteoporosis in both sexes and loss of menstruation in women. Both male and female athletes of all ages can suffer RED-S and it tends to be exacerbated by the perfectionism that is often a character trait – some would say must be a character trait – of elite athletes.

Food can have many uses. Recovery, repair and fuelling are all basic functions for the high-performing cyclist, but the flip side is that we may also use food as a reward or a punishment, or to counter boredom or stress. To be a top athlete you need self-discipline and dedication, and focusing on what you eat is one aspect – one *important* aspect – of that, but for some, focus can tip over into obsession. Constantly thinking or talking about food or frequently missing meals are good indicators that your mindset around food could be better, and if you take an honest look at yourself and think that your relationship with food is not a positive, balanced one, then please seek professional advice from a registered dietician.

If you have an unsuccessful training session or under-perform in a race, don't put that performance down to your diet and react by not eating at all, but equally, don't attempt to deal with your frustration by mainlining chocolate. There's no quick fix, but my mantra is always that you can only race as well as you train, and you can only train well if you're putting enough fuel in the tank for the journey.

So, to summarise: calculate your nutritional needs carefully, cultivate a positive relationship with food, don't pack a family picnic in your back pocket, binge on boxsets and not post-ride banquets, stick to the straight and narrow, but don't go round the bend if you occasionally drift off-track. Have I made myself clear?!

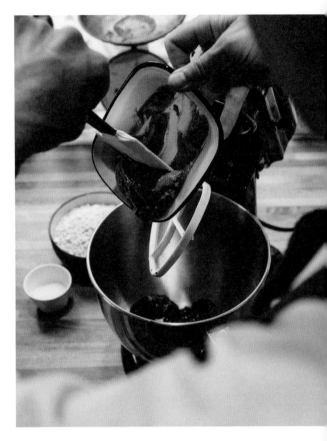

Fresh and delicious meals can be made with surprisingly few ingredients in no time. Invest in some time-saving kitchen appliances – they are a godsend for hungry cyclists in a hurry.

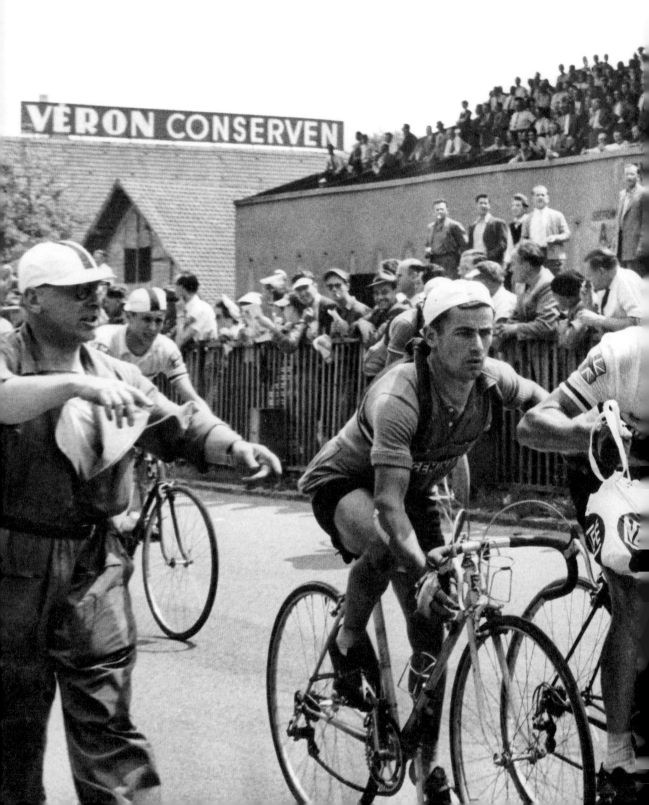

British rider Bob Maitland picks up a bag of provisions during the 1955 Tour de France. In the 1950s a musette typically contained fruit, sandwiches and some sugar lumps.

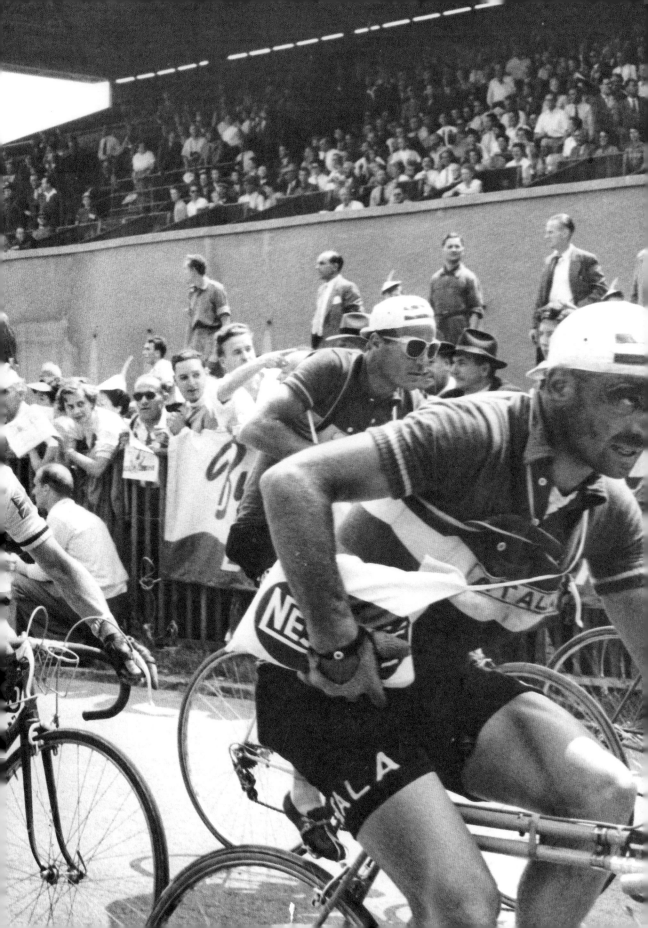

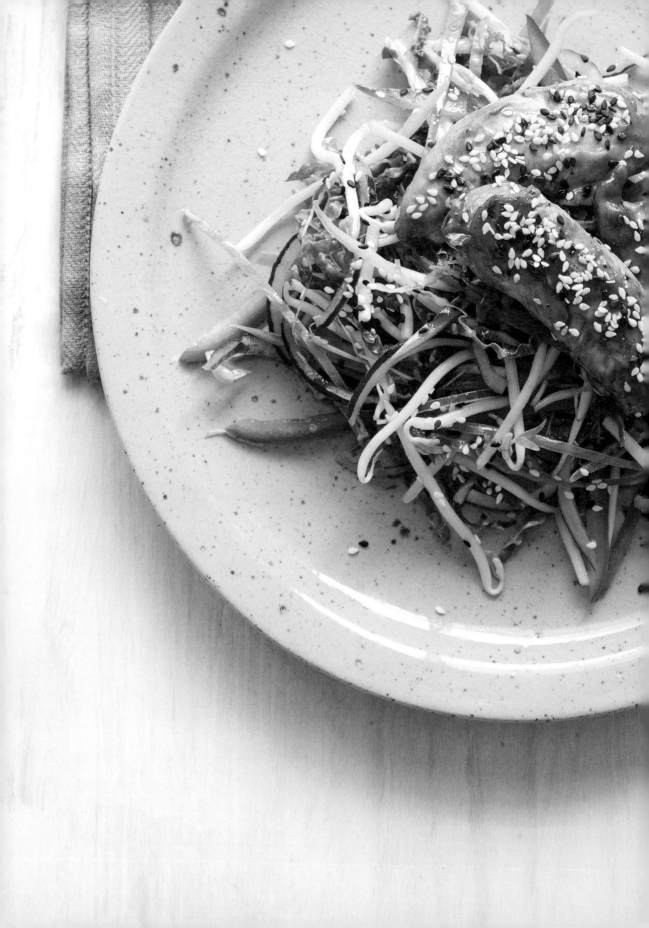

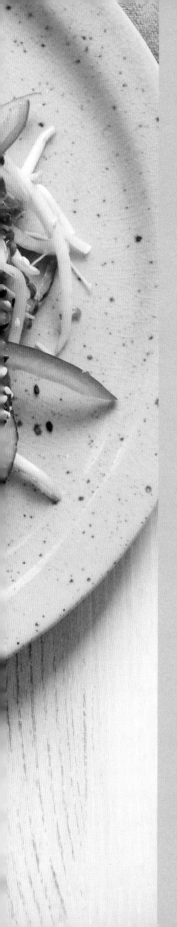

Medium days: Balanced middle-of-the-pack meals

I'm not really a 'vanilla' type of guy. No one's ever accused me of being 'wishy-washy' and 'all or nothing' tends to be my default setting, which is perhaps why I find medium days quite a challenge. I admit I'm not great at moderation, but I suspect I'm not the only one, because a certain amount of obsessiveness is part of what makes us successful cyclists. However, there are times when we all need to give ourselves a break, so sit up and relax a bit – just not too much.

The balance of carbs and protein in my Russian salad with smoked salmon (*see* p. 134) is great after a ride on a gorgeous summer's day that leaves you feeling nicely tired, but not shattered. The Throwback salad Savoyard (*see* p. 137) is another good one for when you get home from that kind of trip out, and I'd suggest packing a 'Wonder Woman' bar (*see* p. 143) for when you take a breather and hop off the bike to enjoy the scenery. They're definitely moreish, but don't be tempted to take two – remember, everything in moderation.

Cheeky cherry breakfast muffins

Easiest recipe you will find – it will take you longer to weigh out the ingredients than to make the actual muffins. Simple and incredibly tasty!

Makes 8 good-sized muffins (snack-size)

1 ripe banana, peeled

300 g (11 oz) frozen cherries

2 free-range eggs

110 g (3½ oz) demerara sugar

125 ml (½ cup) almond milk

110 g (3½ oz) butter, melted

300 g (11 oz) self-raising flour

2 teaspoons cinammon

1 tablespoon poppy seeds

butter to grease

1 teaspoon brown sugar and 1 teaspoon cinnamon, mixed for dusting

1 tablespoon flaked almonds

Nutrition per serving (per muffin):
Energy: 369 kcal
Total carbohydrate: 50 g (of which sugars: 22 g)
Fat: 15 g (of which saturates: 7.9 g)
Fibre: 3.5 g | Protein: 6.9 g | Salt: 0.42 g

LOW-KCAL | MEDIUM-CARB | LOW-PROTEIN

1. Preheat the oven to 180°C/350°F/Gas 4. In the bowl of a food processor blend the banana and half the frozen cherries. Add the eggs, sugar, milk and melted butter, then gradually add the flour, cinnamon and the poppy seeds.

2. Gently stir through the remaining cherries. Spoon the mixture into 8 well-greased muffin moulds, top with the cinnamon and brown sugar mix and sprinkle on the flaked almonds.

3. Bake in the centre of the oven for about 12–14 minutes until golden brown. Transfer to a wire rack to cool.

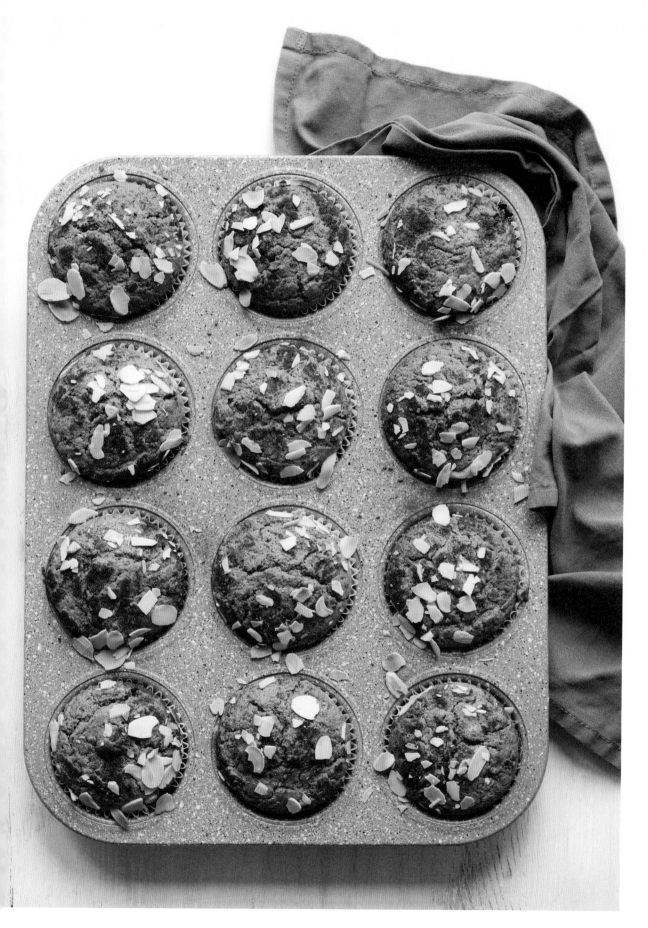

Cherry coconut granola bars

Really tasty and quite addictive, this mix would also work crumbled into yoghurt for a cunning dessert. The bars can be stored in an airtight container for up to 4 days – if they last that long!

**Makes about 16 x 56 g (2 oz) bars
(if you don't eat all the wee bits
when cutting!)
(snack-size)**

butter to grease

200 g (7 oz) rolled oats

30 g (1¼ oz) vanilla protein powder

4 teaspoons desiccated coconut

100 g (3½ oz) chopped glacé Morello cherries

½ teaspoon pink Himalayan salt

145 g (5 oz) crunchy nut butter

180 g (6 oz) maple syrup

2 free-range eggs

1 teaspoon vanilla extract

100 g (3½ oz) white chocolate, chopped

Nutrition per serving:
Energy: 212 kcal
Total carbohydrate: 24 g (of which sugars: 13 g)
Fat: 9.1 g (of which saturates: 2.5 g)
Fibre: 2.9 g | Protein: 6.4 g | Salt: 0.34 g

MEDIUM-KCAL | MEDIUM-CARB | LOW-PROTEIN

1. Preheat the oven to 180°C/350°F/Gas 4. Meanwhile, lightly grease a 20 x 20 cm (8 x 8 in) baking tin.

2. In a large bowl, mix together the oats, protein powder, coconut, chopped cherries and salt.

3. In a separate bowl, combine the crunchy nut butter, maple syrup, eggs and vanilla extract.

4. Transfer wet ingredients to the dry mixture. Mix until oats are well coated before adding the white chocolate.

5. Transfer the mixture to the baking tin and smooth with a palette knife. Place on the middle shelf of the oven and bake for 20 minutes.

6. Allow to cool in the tin for 20–30 minutes before cutting into bars.

Bonzer breakfast burrito

A bit of a change for breakfast, this dish is best cooked and eaten immediately.

Makes 2

2 teaspoons olive oil

½ green pepper, deseeded and finely sliced

½ red onion, peeled and diced

80 g (3 oz) refried beans

10 cherry tomatoes, halved

sea salt and freshly ground black pepper

1 medium avocado, halved, flesh removed, pitted and sliced

2 tortilla wraps

4 free-range eggs

1 tablespoon milk

Nutrition per serving:
Energy: 566 kcal
Total carbohydrate: 39 g (of which sugars: 6.1 g)
Fat: 33 g (of which saturates: 8.1 g)
Fibre: 9.7 g | Protein: 24 g | Salt: 1.6 g

MEDIUM-KCAL | MEDIUM-CARB | HIGH-PROTEIN

1. Preheat the grill to low heat. Heat 1 teaspoon of the olive oil in a large sauté pan set over a medium heat. Add the pepper and onion and fry for 3 minutes, then add the beans and cook for a further 2 minutes. Now add the tomatoes and cook for a further 2 minutes. Season and set aside – cover to keep warm.

2. Prepare your avocado. Slice in half, remove the stone and flesh, then cut the flesh into slices.

3. Toast your wraps for 1 minute each side and keep warm.

4. Whisk the eggs in a bowl with the milk; season well. Heat the remaining olive oil in a small frying pan and cook the eggs over a low heat for 1–2 minutes, stirring constantly until just set.

5. Build your burrito quickly: place peppers and onion, beans, tomatoes, avocado and scrambled eggs in the middle of a toasted wrap and roll up. Eat straight away!

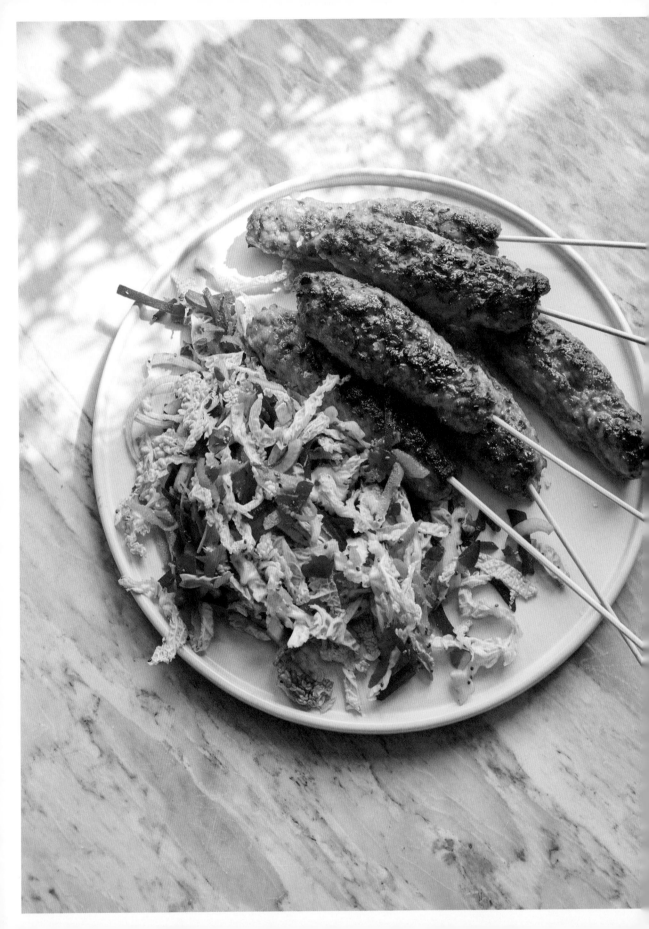

Kofta-style turkey and ghetto slaw

The perfect meal for a lower training load kind of day, this is a great way of serving minced meat. I have used turkey, but you could use pork or beef. The slaw is an ace way to use up any leftover veggies – the acidity of the beetroot and the spice of the chilli sauce cut through the veg.

Serves 2 with a portion left over for lunch the next day

500 g (1 lb 2 oz) minced turkey breast

3 tablespoons plain flour

1 free-range egg

1 teaspoon chopped chilli

1 teaspoon chopped garlic

2 teaspoon spices (BBQ or Cajun work well)

1 dessertspoon tomato purée

good pinch of sea salt and freshly ground black pepper

1 tablespoon olive oil for frying

green salad to serve

Ghetto slaw

2 carrots, trimmed, peeled and grated

180 g (6 oz) pickled beetroot (most supermarkets do really tasty ones in the veg section)

½ Savoy cabbage, sliced

1 onion, peeled and finely sliced

2 tablespoons sweet chilli sauce

1 teaspoon chia seeds

Nutrition per serving:
Energy: 494 kcal
Total carbohydrate: 42 g (of which sugars: 25 g)
Fat: 11 g (of which saturates: 2.5 g)
Fibre: 11 g | Protein: 50 g | Salt: 0.95 g

MEDIUM-KCAL | MEDIUM-CARB | HIGH-PROTEIN

1. For the koftas, mix together all ingredients with the exception of the olive oil. With your hands, shape into 8 large 'sausage' shapes and then mould on to skewers. If your mix is still quite wet, roll in a little flour when moulding. Transfer to a plate and refrigerate for 15 minutes to set.

2. Meanwhile, make the slaw by mixing all the ingredients together in a bowl, cover with a tea towel and set aside.

3. To cook the meat, preheat a large sauté pan, add the olive oil and, once heated, fry the koftas for 7–8 minutes over a low to medium heat, turning frequently.

4. Once cooked, serve with the slaw and some green salad if you need to get your greens in – and then feel fully self-righteous!

Russian salad with smoked salmon

This classic recipe can be made up in advance and is the ideal post-ride meal on a warm summer's day.

Serves 2

100 g (3½ oz) frozen peas

150 g (5 oz) carrots (peeled weight)

100 g (3½ oz) turnip or swede (peeled weight)

150 g (5 oz) potatoes (peeled weight)

1 tablespoon chopped capers

1 tablespoon chopped gherkins

4 anchovies, chopped

2 tablespoons low-calorie mayonnaise

sea salt and freshly ground black pepper

240 g (9 oz) smoked salmon and a bag of mixed salad leaves to serve

Nutrition per serving:
Energy: 467 kcal
Total carbohydrate: 31 g (of which sugars: 15 g)
Fat: 20 g (of which saturates: 3.5 g)
Fibre: 10 g | Protein: 36 g | Salt: 5.2 g

MEDIUM-KCAL | LOW-CARB | LOW-PROTEIN

1. Defrost the peas. Meanwhile, dice all the vegetables and simmer in boiling salted water until they still have a wee bit of bite (al dente), then drain well.

2. In a large bowl, combine the vegetables with the capers, gherkins, anchovies and mayonnaise.

3. Adjust the seasoning and serve with the smoked salmon and salad leaves.

Banging broth of chicken, mushroom and ginger

Clean oriental flavours, ideal for easier days on the bike. This light and tasty broth is really simple, but a lot comes down to the quality of the stock used. I would normally say that life is too short to make your own chicken stock, but now is the time to ignore my usual advice. The base broth mix (steps 1–2) can easily be made up in advance, leaving you to cook the pork, mushrooms and green bits when required.

Serves 2

750 ml (3 cups) chicken stock (ideally homemade)

35 g (1½ oz) chopped fresh ginger, grated

3 teaspoons finely chopped lemongrass

1 tablespoon Thai fish sauce

1 tablespoon soy sauce

sea salt and freshly ground black pepper

300 g (11 oz) pork loin, cut into strips

1 green pepper, deseeded and finely sliced

1 red onion, peeled and finely sliced

300 g (11 oz) mixed mushrooms (shiitake, oyster, chestnut all work well), chopped

150 g (5 oz) mix of pak choi and Chinese cabbage, sliced

100 g (3½ oz) edamame beans

1 bunch coriander, chopped

1. To a large saucepan, add the chicken stock, ginger and lemongrass. Simmer for 30 minutes and then add the fish sauce and soy sauce. Check the seasoning and set aside.

2. When ready to serve, simmer the stock and add the pork. Simmer for 4 minutes.

3. Add the pepper, onion and mushrooms. Simmer for a further 2 minutes.

4. To retain freshness, stir in the pak choi, Chinese cabbage, edamame beans and coriander at the end of the cooking time and simmer for a final 2 minutes. Check the seasoning again and then serve.

Nutrition per serving:
Energy: 598 kcal
Total carbohydrate: 24 g (of which sugars: 14 g)
Fat: 31 g (of which saturates: 10 g)
Fibre: 5.3 g | Protein: 52 g | Salt: 5 g

MEDIUM-KCAL | LOW-CARB | HIGH-PROTEIN

Glazed gnocchi, roasted red pepper, tomato and smoked chorizo

This dish can be made up in advance and popped in the oven when you get in the door. Smoked or spicy chorizo? That is the question…

Serves 2 with portion left for lunch

400 g (14 oz) fresh gnocchi

1 small onion, peeled and finely chopped

1 teaspoon chopped garlic

1 teaspoon chopped red chilli

100 g (3½ oz) smoked chorizo, diced

2 red peppers, deseeded and sliced

1 teaspoon smoked paprika

500 g (1 lb 2 oz) passata

sea salt and freshly ground black pepper

30 g (1¼ oz) grated Parmesan

1 bunch of basil, finely chopped, to finish

Nutrition per serving:
Energy: 510 kcal
Total carbohydrate: 67 g (of which sugars: 21 g)
Fat: 15 g (of which saturates: 6.1 g)
Fibre: 7.8 g | Protein: 21 g | Salt: 2.6 g

MEDIUM-KCAL | MEDIUM-CARB | HIGH-PROTEIN

1. Preheat the oven to 180°C/350°F/Gas 4. Cook the gnocchi for 90 seconds in boiling salted water, strain well and set aside.

2. To a medium sauté pan placed over a low to medium heat, add the onion, garlic, chilli, chorizo and peppers (you don't need to add any oil as the fat in the chorizo will render down). Cook slowly for 10 minutes.

3. Stir in the smoked paprika and passata and simmer for 5 minutes. Adjust the seasoning and then stir in the cooked gnocchi.

4. Transfer the mixture to an ovenproof dish, top with Parmesan and bake in the centre of the oven for 10 minutes.

5. Finish off by sprinkling the chopped basil over the top just before serving.

Throwback salad Savoyard

It's quite unusual to have such a substantial filling salad. This is great for a post-ride meal in summer. For me it's a bit of a throwback dish as I spent a few years working in the Alps as a young chef and this was a staple on many local menus (the last year I worked in the Alps was Miguel Indurain's fifth Tour de France win and I followed the race around the high mountains, spectating).

Adding bacon and cheese to anything makes it taste amazing… chef fact! Note: the dressing makes enough for 4 people so keep the rest covered in the fridge for another time. It will last for up to 4 weeks. The nutritional info below is calculated using a drizzle of dressing per serving.

Serves 2

100 g (3½ oz) diced smoked back bacon

100 g (3½ oz) Gruyère cheese (being a purist, you would try to use Comté or Beaufort)

200 g (7 oz) cooked new potatoes

1 slice bread for croutons

1 teaspoon olive oil

25 g (1 oz) walnuts

1 large frisée salad, roughly chopped or a large bag of mixed salad leaves to serve

Dressing

1 teaspoon Dijon mustard

2 tablespoons white wine vinegar

3 tablespoons extra virgin olive oil

2 tablespoons water

Nutrition per serving:
Energy: 584 kcal
Total carbohydrate: 22 g of which sugars): 4.3 g)
Fat: 41 g (of which saturates: 16 g)
Fibre: 5.3 g | Protein: 28 g | Salt: 2.5 g

MEDIUM-KCAL | LOW-CARB | HIGH-PROTEIN

1. Preheat the grill to medium. Arrange the bacon on a baking sheet and grill until crispy, then set aside.

2. Dice up your cheese and new potatoes, then set aside.

3. To make the croutons, dice the bread and combine in a bowl with the olive oil. Warm a non-stick pan over a low heat and cook until the croutons are golden brown.

4. Prepare the salad dressing by mixing the mustard with the white wine vinegar in a bowl. Slowly whisk in the oil and water.

5. To serve, combine all the salad ingredients together in a large bowl and then spoon over the dressing.

Teriyaki chicken, beansprouts, sweet chilli and pepper salad

For when calorie and carb intake can be less due to a reduced training load, this crunchy salad makes a perfect packed lunch – all the ingredients are readily available and it's very quick to knock together. If you have vegan tendencies, it would work just as well with tofu instead of chicken – follow the same method of grilling until sticky. It's also simple to carb up – cook some rice noodles and away you go!

Serves 3 – 2 mains and a fight for leftovers for lunch the next day!

500 g (1 lb 2 oz) chicken mini fillets

2 tablespoons Teriyaki marinade (available from supermarkets)

1 teaspoon sesame oil

150 g (5 oz) Savoy cabbage, finely sliced

300 g (11 oz) beansprouts

1 small red onion, peeled and finely sliced

1 red pepper, deseeded and finely sliced

100 g (3½ oz) mangetout, finely sliced

squeeze of lime juice

2 tablespoons light soy sauce

2 tablespoons sweet chilli sauce

small bunch of coriander, chopped

1 teaspoon of sesame seeds, mix of black and white

Nutrition per serving:
Energy: 402 kcal
Total carbohydrate: 23 g (of which sugars: 19 g)
Fat: 7.1 g (of which saturates: 1.2 g)
Fibre: 5.9 g | Protein: 58 g | Salt: 2.6 g

MEDIUM-KCAL | LOW-CARB | HIGH-PROTEIN

1. Preheat a grill to medium heat. Combine the chicken, Teriyaki marinade and sesame oil with your hands on a non-stick baking tray. Grill for 6–8 minutes, turning, until the chicken is cooked and a wee bit sticky, then allow to cool.

2. In a large bowl, mix together all the vegetables, then stir in the lime juice, soy sauce and sweet chilli sauce.

3. At the last minute add the coriander and then top with the cooked chicken and sesame seeds.

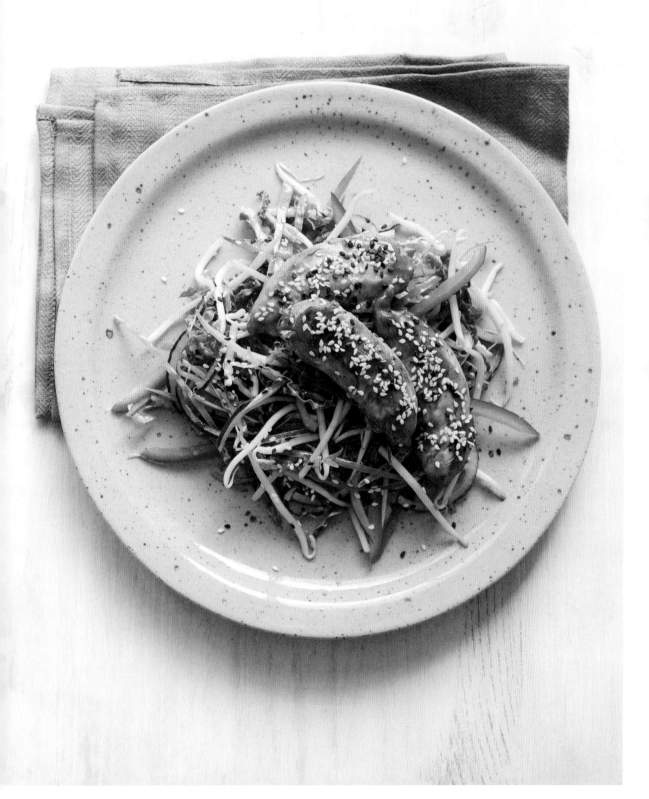

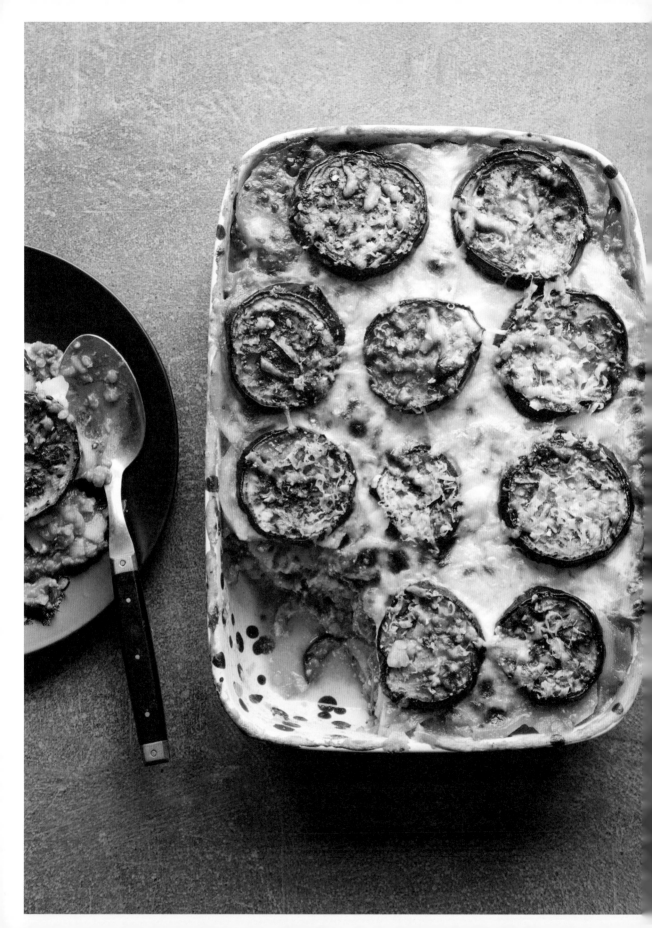

Auntie Mo's moussaka

Perhaps one of my earliest food memories was my Auntie Mo making up what seemed like the most luxurious and exotic-sounding dish ever… moussaka! As an eight-year-old, I'd never even seen an aubergine, let alone tasted one.

There are three parts to this dish – the meaty bit, the veg bit and the white sauce. Also, please read the aubergine prep carefully. Traditionally, moussaka is made using minced lamb, but you can also make it with beef or to 'lean it up', use turkey breast mince if you fancy it.

Serves 4

500 g (1 lb 2 oz) Stretch lentil mince (*see* p. 159)

good pinch of cinnamon

250 g (9 oz) passata

sea salt and freshly ground black pepper

600 g (1¼ lb) Maris piper potatoes (peeled weight)

2 medium aubergines

good pinch of salt

1 tablespoon olive oil

'Cowboy' white sauce

500 ml (2 cups) milk

25 g (1 oz) butter

4 teaspoons cornflour

3 tablespoons cold water

40 g (1½ oz) grated Parmesan

green salad to serve

Nutrition per serving:
Energy: 538 kcal
Total carbohydrate: 61 g (of which sugars: 17 g)
Fat: 17 g (of which saturates: 8.2 g)
Fibre: 8.5 g | Protein: 29 g | Salt: 1.1 g

MEDIUM-KCAL | MEDIUM-CARB | HIGH-PROTEIN

1. First, make the Bolognese sauce and stir in the cinnamon and passata. Season well and set aside.

2. Meanwhile, slice the potatoes thinly and boil lightly in salted water for 5 minutes, then strain and set aside.

3. Now make the white sauce with this quick and easy/cowboy method. Gently simmer the milk and butter in a saucepan. In a bowl, make a paste with the cornflour and water. Whisk into the simmering milk/butter a little at a time until the sauce thickens, being careful not to catch the bottom of the pan. Stir in half the Parmesan and check the seasoning.

4. Aubergines… Normally, cooking aubergines is savage as they soak up oil like a sponge. Here's what I suggest: slice the aubergines thinly and sprinkle on some salt, leave for 15 minutes and then brush with olive oil. Then either grill under a very hot grill for 2–3 minutes or blow-torch until lightly charred.

5. Preheat the oven to 190°C/375°F/Gas 5. Meanwhile, take a 20 x 20 cm (8 x 8 in) ovenproof dish. Layer up the Bolognese, potatoes, 'cowboy' white sauce, then the aubergines, Bolognese, potatoes, white sauce, aubergines and white sauce. Sprinkle the remaining Parmesan over the top and bake in the oven for 30 minutes. Serve with a green salad.

Posh poached eggs

Try this as a lush light lunch or evening meal. The key here is poaching the eggs – a little bit of technique is required but once mastered, you can't go wrong. I suggest you read the recipe twice as timing is crucial. If possible, buy eggs from your local farm shop – they are always much better than any supermarket varieties.

This dish also requires a bit of multitasking as you will need to cook the mushroom mix while poaching the eggs and making toast. Best make sure you're not on Instagram at the same time!

Serves 1

25 g (1 oz) unsalted butter

125 g (4 oz) mixed wild mushrooms or chestnut mushrooms

sea salt and freshly ground black pepper

80 g (3 oz) baby spinach leaves

75 g (3 oz) chunk of sourdough

Poached eggs

1 tablespoon white vinegar

1 teaspoon salt

2 large free-range eggs

Nutrition per serving:
Energy: 617 kcal
Total carbohydrate: 46 g (of which sugars: 4.3 g)
Fat: 34 g (of which saturates: 17 g)
Fibre: 5.4 g | Protein: 30 g | Salt: 1.5 g

HIGH-KCAL | MEDIUM-CARB | HIGH-PROTEIN

1. Preheat a sauté pan, add the butter and quickly fry the mushrooms, 2–3 minutes. Season well, then add the spinach and cook for 30 seconds over a high heat. Transfer the mixture to a colander to strain off any excess liquid.

2. While the mushroom mix is cooking, cook the poached eggs (see below) and toast the sourdough once the eggs are cooking.

3. Tip the spinach and mushroom mix on to the toast, then top with the poached eggs and serve immediately.

Perfect poached eggs

1. Three-quarter fill a medium saucepan with hot water and set over the heat. Add the vinegar and the salt and bring to the boil.

2. Crack the eggs into a small bowl, being extra careful not to break the yolks.

3. Whisk the cooking water to form a 'whirlpool' effect and while the water is still spinning, gently pour in the eggs into the centre.

4. Bring the water back up to the boil and simmer gently for 2–3 minutes until cooked but still soft to the touch.

5. Remove the eggs from the water with a slotted spoon, strain well and serve as above.

'Wonder Woman' bars

These bars are high in iron and also provide a decent hit of vitamin C. Lemon and cherry are a true classic flavour profile, and while you'll have to hunt down some specialist ingredients it's well worth the effort. Camu camu is a tiny berry found in the heart of the Amazon rainforest. Luckily, you don't need to forage for it there as you will find it dried and powdered in your local health food shop. Store the bars in an airtight container in the fridge for up to 2 weeks.

Makes 20 bars – 46 g (1½ oz) (snack-size)

40 g (1½ oz) blackstrap molasses

250 g (9 oz) medjool dates

½ teaspoon lemon essential oil

4 teaspoons camu camu powder

75 g (3 oz) chia seeds

150 g (5 oz) dried chopped apricots

75 g (3 oz) dried cherries

125 g (4 oz) whole green pistachios

85 g (3¼ oz) puffed quinoa (or use Rice Krispies)

100 g (3½ oz) ground almonds

1. In the bowl of a food processor, blend the molasses, dates, lemon oil, camu camu and chia seeds.

2. Stir in the apricots, cherries, pistachios and puffed quinoa so they retain their lovely texture. Finally, mix in the ground almonds.

3. Tip the mixture into a greaseproof-lined tin 22 x 22 cm (10 x 10 in) and press firmly with your fingertips to flatten smoothly into the tin. Refrigerate for 3 hours until set and then slice into bars.

Nutrition per serving:
Energy: 183 kcal
Total carbohydrate: 21 g (of which sugars: 16 g)
Fat: 7.7 g (of which saturates: 0.8 g)
Fibre: 5.7 g | Protein: 4.9 g | Salt: 0.03 g

MEDIUM-KCAL | MEDIUM-CARB | LOW-PROTEIN

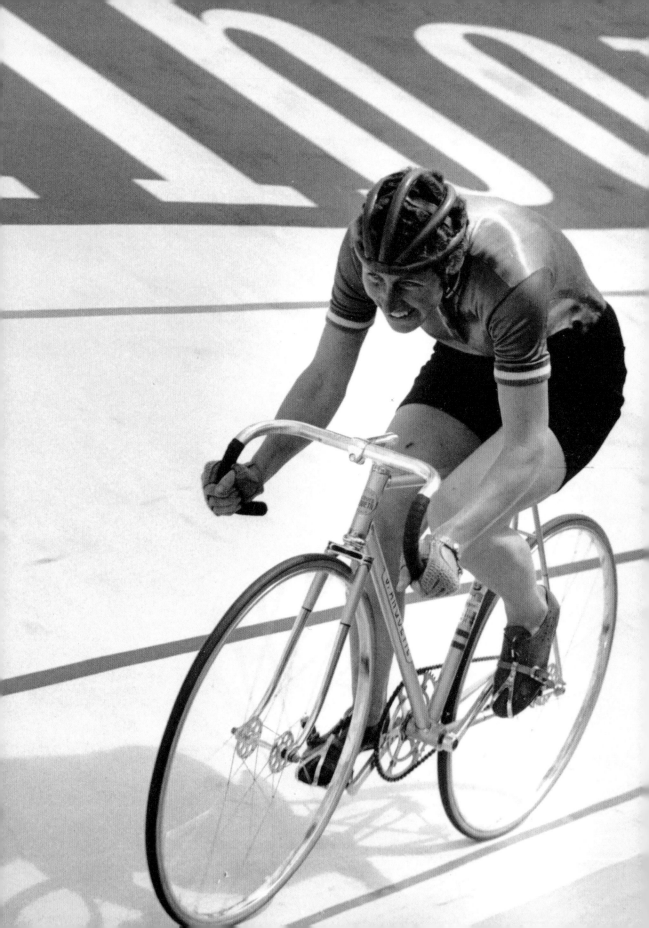

The Long Game

Can you see yourself crossing that line?
Do you burst from the bunch with 20 seconds
to go, or do you haul yourself valiantly up
the last 200 metres, having been on a solo
breakaway? Yes, I know it's what a sports
psychologist would say, but it genuinely
does help to visualise your goals.

Former women's world cycle champion
Beryl Burton digs deep to take the bronze
medal in the 3000 m Pursuit during the
World Cycling Championships in Leicester
in 1970.

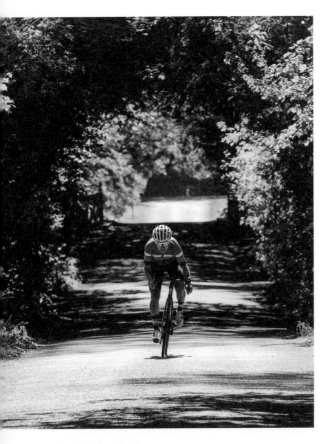

Pre-season is the time to get serious. Aim for slow and steady weight loss as your training intensifies in the 12 weeks of the run-up to race season.

Losing weight is hard work and, frankly, I'm afraid there are no real shortcuts. Crash diets aren't good for you and they're not good for your form either, because when your body goes into starvation mode, it puts a hold on fitness development and locks down fat stores. A crash diet will leave you feeling physically depleted, because your body simply isn't able to adjust to the sharp drop in food intake and your mental health will probably suffer, too.

Every serious cyclist needs to accept that, to a certain extent, their fitness levels and weight will go up and down over the course of the year. In winter, we all need a little more resolve to get on the bike and we crave comfort food. Then, when the pressure is off and training schedules are more relaxed, that's probably the time when we'll really want to treat our taste buds. What you need – and this is very much an ideal, but I promise you it's an achievable ideal – is a plan that matches what you eat to your training programme and delivers slow and steady weight loss over a period of, say, the 12 weeks of the run-up to race season. Alternatively, identify a key event and work back from there.

Studies show that those who hop on the scales regularly do tend to lose more weight over time,[12] probably because the scales present them with an ongoing series of micro-goals, but don't become obsessed with that readout and whatever diet plan you're following, remember your weight can fluctuate hugely on a daily basis. Depletion of glycogen stores and being even slightly dehydrated can give a false weight loss, whereas high-fibre meals – or, for me, gluten – and mistimed bowel movements can result in the scales 'lying' to the tune of a couple of kilos. Fluid retention at certain times during their menstrual cycle can cause women's weight to fluctuate even more. In many ways, you should embrace weight fluctuations, so, for instance, carrying a few kilos extra if you're in an endurance block can be a real advantage, because it gives you an energy reserve to work with.

Nutritional gain

That said, when the time comes to shift those kilos, there are various approaches that can be helpful and nutrient timing is one of them. This is about consuming combinations of nutrients, primarily protein and carbohydrate, before, during and after training sessions. Some people claim nutrient timing can produce quite dramatic improvements in your body composition or proportion of muscle to fat. In fact, some people believe the timing is more crucial than what you actually eat, although I'm a chef so I certainly wouldn't go that far.

To give an example, many experts believe the time after you've exercised is most critical for nutrient timing. In theory, consuming the right ratio of nutrients after a ride or training session not only turns the ignition key for the process of repairing muscles and restoring energy reserves, but turbo-charges it, amplifying its effects on both performance and body composition. The recipes in the Pre-season section (*see* pp. 50-67) will probably be particularly useful to you here.

Periodised nutrition takes this idea further and is about carefully planning your diet over the longer term to complement and enhance certain periods of your training programme. It aims to ensure you get the most out of the hours spent on your bike and there are a few ways you can implement it, as follows.

Carrying a few kilos extra if you're in an endurance block can be a real advantage, because it gives you an energy reserve to work with.

You may not see the results on the scales immediately, but they will materialise eventually and translate into results on the track or road.

Training lows and highs

'Training low' means training with low-carbohydrate availability. As we've touched on previously, one example would be training after you've fasted overnight and before you eat breakfast. Or, if you train twice a day, restricting your carbohydrate intake after the first session means you'll approach the second session with low-carb availability. During a race, your body will be able to tap into your fat stores better, so you'll be able to sustain your performance better. There are some issues to be aware of, though, because training low can increase the risk of illness and injury, or lead to reduced immune function, so it's best to get professional advice on implementing this strategy.

A similar approach is sleeping low, which means training hard later in the day, eating a low-carb meal and then going more or less straight to bed. Because muscle and liver glycogen are likely to be low for several hours while you sleep, this can potentially drive your body to adapt to lower fuel levels overnight. It's important to fuel well the following morning, though, especially if you plan to train hard first thing. This strategy can deliver performance improvements, but it can also impact on the quality of your sleep, so don't do it too often and, again, it's best to get professional advice and monitor your ongoing health. What's more, you don't want to get anything less than eight hours' sleep a night, because studies have shown that reduced sleep can inhibit weight loss.[13]

Training high, on the other hand, means training on full glycogen stores and supplementing these with carbs while you ride. This should promote top-notch performances, particularly if upping your speed is an objective, and reduce fatigue. Training high should also accustom your gut to tolerating the carbohydrate which you need to consume during endurance events. For higher-intensity training, up your carb intake even further, but avoid this for extended periods of time, because if your body becomes too accustomed to a high-carb diet, it will stop adapting and your weight loss will stop as well.

I recommend doing some detailed research into each of the approaches I've outlined here (the TrainingPeaks platform [www.trainingpeaks. com] has some useful resources), maybe getting some professional advice, working out which tactic delivers the maximum impact for you as a rider and matching that up with recipes from the different sections in this book. The key here is to be strategic and to deploy nutrition in conjunction with your training programme.

I'm only human and you're only human, too, so there are always times when you should cut yourself some slack, but I do my utmost to practise what I preach, because I know it works. You may not see the results on the scales immediately, but they will materialise eventually and translate into results on the track or road. Remember, you're in this for the long haul, so persevere and be patient – but don't forget to enjoy the ride!

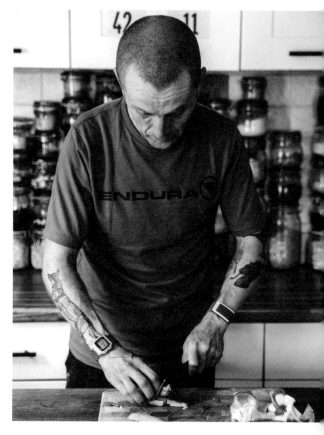

Some easy-to-learn culinary skills can help you produce a range of appetising dishes full of flavour and texture, which can boost energy levels, aid muscle recovery and lead to better performances.

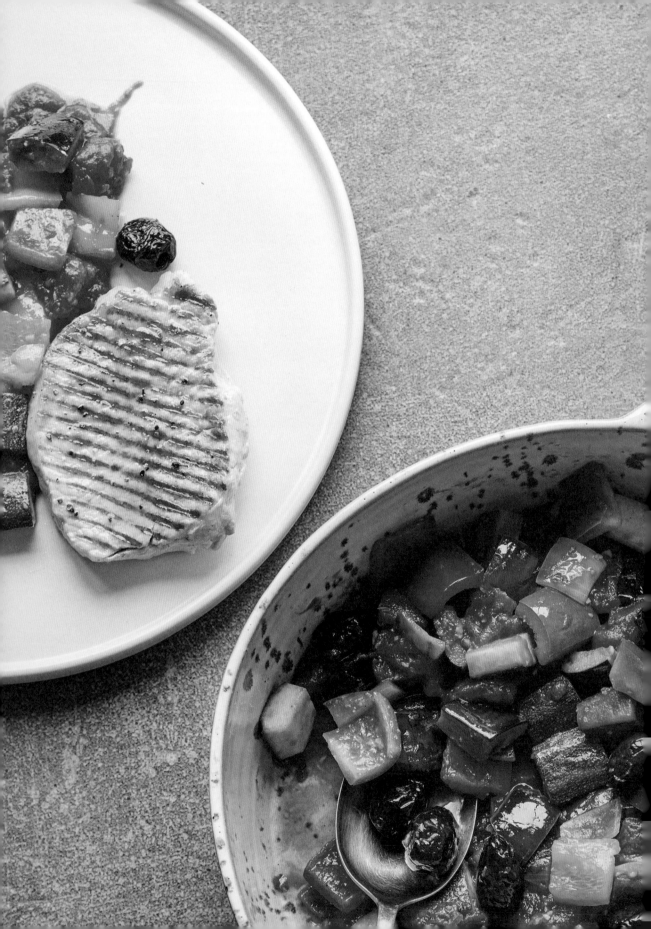

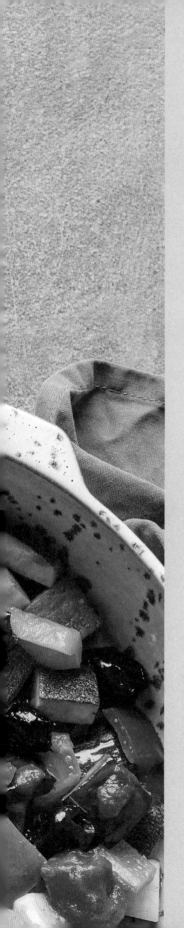

Hard days: Fuelling the machine

OK, this section is all about fuelling the machine, so it's full gas on both the carbs and the protein to boost energy and recovery. However, I promise you there's no let up on the strong flavour and texture combos. Turkey 'Keith Reynolds' (*see* p. 164) is always popular. Basically, turkey steaks with a coriander pesto and veg slaw, it was named for British Cycling's logistics manager (also a great pro back in the day). The Smoked paprika, tomato and thyme meatballs (*see* p. 168) go down well every time, too, and the Stretch lentil and beef Bolognese (*see* p. 159) isn't half bad either! Quality food for a quality performance on the bike – that sums it up.

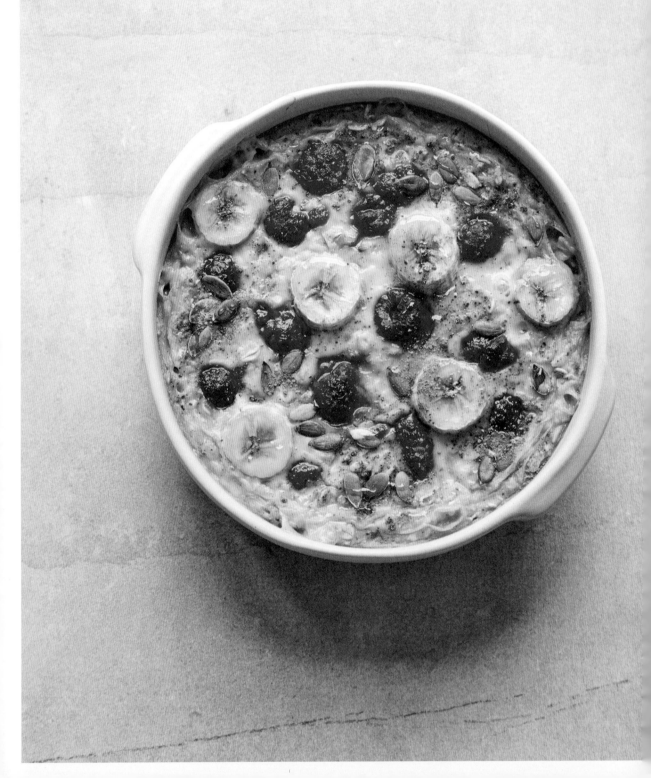

Baked oats recipes

Baking oats… Surely this is just porridge with fancy pants on? Nope, there's something quite magical about a slightly crunchy topping with oats and scalding hot fruit! The base recipe and technique are the starting point and once you have that mastered, you can freestyle flavour profiles. Here are three of my favourites…

Raspberry-banana ripple-baked oats

Reminiscent of old-school ice cream van flavours and so luxurious it almost feels like dessert… but don't be having a scoop of vanilla ice cream with it for breakfast!

Serves 2

100 g (3½ oz) oats

300 ml (1¼ cups) boiling water

2 bananas, peeled

80 g (3 oz) frozen raspberries

25 g (1 oz) almonds, skin-on, crushed

1 teaspoon cinnamon

1 teaspoon vanilla extract

2 tablespoons honey

200 ml (¾ cup) almond milk

1 tablespoon pumpkin seeds

Nutrition per serving:
Energy: 502 kcal
Total carbohydrate: 72 g (of which sugars: 37 g)
Fat: 14 g (of which saturates: 1.7 g)
Fibre: 11 g | Protein: 13 g | Salt: 0.14 g

MEDIUM-KCAL | HIGH-CARB | MEDIUM-PROTEIN

1. Preheat the oven to 180°C/350°F/Gas 4. Meanwhile, place the oats in a bowl and cover with boiling water, just so the top of the oats is covered. Soak for 10 minutes until softened. Not a second more.

2. Slice 1 banana and mash the other in a bowl with a fork.

3. Stir through the oats the mashed banana, raspberries, almonds, cinnamon, vanilla, half the honey and the almond milk.

4. Pour the mixture into an ovenproof dish and top with sliced banana. Spoon over the remaining honey and the pumpkin seeds.

5. Place in the centre of the oven and bake for 20–25 minutes until golden brown. When cooked, allow it to sit for 10 minutes as it will be way too hot to eat.

Cherry 'baked well' oats

Cherry and almond… mmm! What's not to like about this all-time classic flavour profile? Frozen cherries work a treat as preparing and removing the stones from fresh cherries can be a pain. This breakfast is so tasty it could almost be a dessert. Now that's got me thinking… Could we have custard for breakfast too?

Serves 2

100 g (3½ oz) rolled oats

300 ml (1¼ cups) boiling water

200 ml (¾ cup) vanilla soya milk

1 tablespoon honey

1 ripe banana, peeled and mashed

80 g (3 oz) frozen cherries

40 g (1½ oz) cherry concentrate

a few drops of almond extract, if liked

1 tablespoon ground almonds

1 teaspoon flaked almonds

Nutrition per serving:
Energy: 498 kcal
Total carbohydrate: 76 g (of which sugars: 38 g)
Fat: 13 g (of which saturates: 1.6 g)
Fibre: 7.6 g | Protein: 14 g | Salt: 0.16 g

MEDIUM-KCAL | HIGH-CARB | MEDIUM-PROTEIN

1. Preheat the oven to 190°C/375°F/Gas 5. Place the oats in a heatproof dish, pour over the boiling water and leave for 10 minutes. Not a second more.

2. Stir in the vanilla soya milk, honey, mashed banana, half of the frozen cherries, cherry concentrate, almond extract if using and the ground almonds.

3. Make a fancy pants arrangement of the rest of the cherries and flaked almonds on the top (Instagram purposes only) and bake in the centre of the oven for 20–25 minutes. If feeling 'cheffy', glaze under a hot grill for a crispy topping

4. Leave it to sit for 10 minutes before eating so that you don't melt your tongue!

Apple strudel flavour baked oats

High in carbs so ideal for a hardcore weekend ride. Could this be the best flavour profile ever? Also, think about this one: dessert the night before a big ride? Why not add a scoop of vanilla ice cream? A bit more work is required as you need to make an apple purée in advance – make sure you use cooking apples for this as they will break down nicely.

Serves 2

100 g (3½ oz) rolled oats

300 ml (1¼ cups) boiling water

185 ml (¾ cup) oat milk

1 ripe banana, peeled and mashed

1 teaspoon cinnamon

1 teaspoon vanilla extract

50 g (2 oz) raisins

1 cored, peeled and sliced eating apple for the topping

1 tablespoon crushed pecans

1 tablespoon honey

Purée

200 g (7 oz) Bramley apples, peeled, cored and diced

2 tablespoons brown sugar

4 tablespoons water

squeeze of lemon

1. Preheat the oven to 190°C/375°F/Gas 5.

2. First, make the purée. Place the diced apple, brown sugar, water and lemon juice in a saucepan. Stir and cook over a medium heat until softened, about 10 minutes.

3. Place the oats in an ovenproof dish. Pour over the boiling water and leave for 10 minutes, not a second more. Stir in the oat milk, mashed banana, apple purée, cinnamon, vanilla and raisins.

4. Arrange sliced apple and crushed pecans on the top and drizzle over the honey. Bake in the centre of the oven for 20–25 minutes. If you want to crisp it up, flash it briefly under the grill.

5. Wait 10 minutes before tucking in as it will be scalding hot.

Nutrition per serving:
Energy: 646 kcal
Total carbohydrate: 114 g (of which sugars: 77 g)
Fat: 14 g (of which saturates: 1.6 g)
Fibre: 11 g | Protein: 10 g | Salt: 0.16 g

HIGH-KCAL | HIGH-CARB | LOW-PROTEIN

Tikka 'tattie scones' with coconut lentil dahl

A post-hard training ride meal at its finest, this is nostalgia food of the highest order. As a lad, a weekly treat was my Granny's classic 'tattie scone'. This technique was taught to me at an early age and I've taken the old classic and added an Indian twist – works rather well, I think. I'm not too sure what Granny would have made of a lentil dahl, mind you!

Makes 4 portions

500 g (1 lb 2 oz) potatoes (cooked and mashed weight, Desirée works best)

30 g (1¼ oz) butter, melted (plus extra for frying)

½ teaspoon salt

1 medium free-range egg

125 g (4 oz) plain flour (plus a little extra for rolling out)

½ teaspoon turmeric

1 teaspoon tikka curry powder

1 teaspoon black onion seeds

1 teaspoon baking powder

sea salt and freshly ground black pepper

Coconut dahl

1 tablespoon olive oil

1 small onion, peeled and diced

1 tablespoon mild Madras curry powder

1 teaspoon chopped chilli

1 teaspoon chopped garlic

250 g (9 oz) red lentils

400 ml (1½ cups) coconut milk

200 ml (¾ cup) vegetable stock

sea salt and freshly ground black pepper

small bunch of coriander, chopped

1. First, make the dahl. Heat the olive oil in a saucepan, add the onion and fry gently for 4–5 minutes over a low heat.

2. Next, add the curry powder, chilli and garlic and cook for a further 3 minutes.

3. Stir in the lentils, coconut milk and stock. Simmer gently over a low heat for 25–30 minutes, stirring every so often, being careful not to burn the bottom of the pan. When the mix is cooked down, season well, add the coriander and set aside.

4. The second job is to make the scones. Combine the mashed potatoes, butter, salt, egg, flour, turmeric, tikka curry powder, black onion seeds and baking powder in a large mixing bowl. Season well, but be careful not to overwork.

5. On a floured surface, use a rolling pin to roll out the scone dough to a 5 mm (¼ in) thickness. Cut out rounds using an 8 cm (3½ in) diameter pastry cutter (you will get 8–10 scones).

6. Heat a knob of butter in a large frying pan and cook the tattie scones for 3–4 minutes each side until nicely browned. You can keep them warm in the oven while you cook the rest of the batch. Serve the warm scones (2–3 per person) with the dahl for a fantastic meal!

Nutrition per serving:
Energy: 745 kcal
Total carbohydrate: 87 g (of which sugars: 6.4 g)
Fat: 31 g (of which saturates: 22 g)
Fibre: 8 g | Protein: 25 g | Salt: 2.6 g

HIGH-KCAL | HIGH-CARB | HIGH-PROTEIN

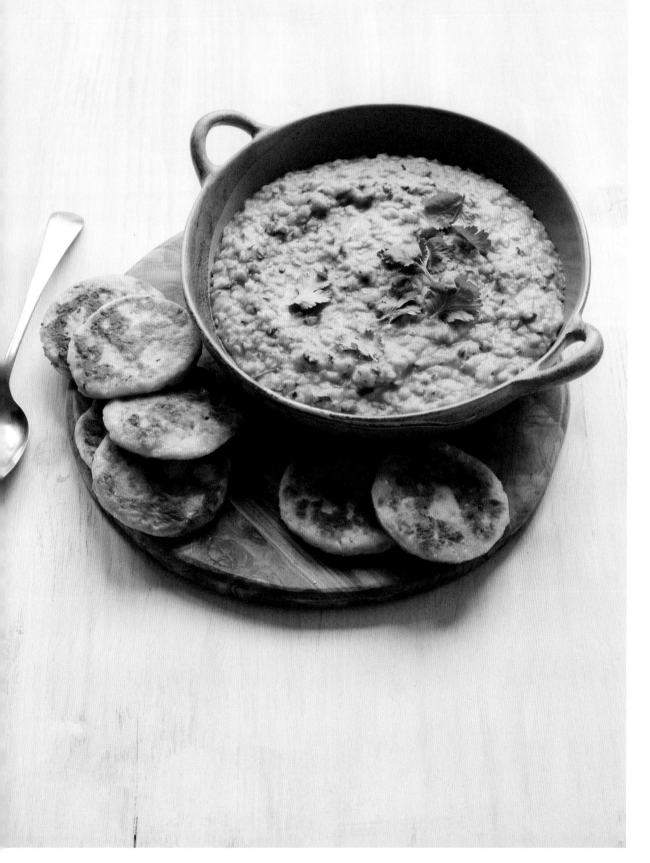

'Meat sweats' breakfast burrito

A big old breakfast, this one – just what you want the morning after an honest day in the saddle. You're guaranteed to be full until lunchtime!

Serves 2

3 chicken sausages

4 smoked back bacon rashers

100 g (3½ oz) black pudding, diced

150 g (5 oz) baked beans

1 teaspoon olive oil

2 large free-range eggs

sea salt and freshly ground black pepper

2 large tortilla wraps

Nutrition per serving:
Energy: 761 kcal
Total carbohydrate: 52 g (of which sugars: 5.4 g)
Fat: 37 g (of which saturates: 13 g)
Fibre: 7.1 g | Protein: 52 g | Salt: 6.4 g

HIGH-KCAL | MEDIUM-CARB | HIGH-PROTEIN

1. Preheat the grill to a medium heat and grill the chicken sausages for 3 minutes on each side. Add the bacon and black pudding and cook for a further 2 minutes each side. Make sure the sausages are cooked through, then slice into thick chunks and keep everything warm under a low grill.

2. Heat the beans in a small saucepan.

3. Heat the olive oil in a small sauté or frying pan. Gently fry the eggs for 3–4 minutes, then season with sea salt and black pepper.

4. Warm your tortilla wraps under the grill.

5. Once everything is ready, place a tortilla wrap on each plate and then artistically arrange everything else on top, cheffy style, or just pile it on and get stuck in!

Stretch upgrades… Like putting wheels on your bike – the same but better!

OK, so this is a great way to make your meat supply go further. No bad news here as it means we eat less meat, plus it's cheaper, with increased fibre and fewer calories – all for the same full-on flavour. Make up a batch of the base Stretch lentil and beef Bolognese, below, and then customise it as you fancy. You can serve it as is with spaghetti for a classic Bolognese; top it with mash and bake for a homely cottage pie (*see* p. 160), or spice it up for a Moroccan mince (*see* p. 161) – three totally different flavour profiles to fuel any type of ride.

Stretch lentil and beef Bolognese

Keep things simple with this classic Bolognese. It's a go-to for when you want to maximise your time on the bike and minimise your time in the kitchen.

Makes 6 decent portions

1 teaspoon olive oil for frying

500 g (1 lb 2 oz) beef mince
(5 per cent fat)

250 g (9 oz) red lentils

1 chicken stock cube (I use Knorr Stock Pots)

650 ml (2½ cups) boiling water

2 small onions, peeled and chopped

2 teaspoons garlic purée

500 g (1 lb 2 oz) passata

sea salt and freshly ground black pepper

dry-weight pasta of your choice (spaghetti or fusilli work well, allow 100 g (3½ oz) per person) to serve

Nutrition per serving (with pasta):
Energy: 646 kcal
Total carbohydrate: 98 g (of which sugars: 9.7 g)
Fat: 6.7 g (of which saturates: 2.2 g)
Fibre: 7.4 g | Protein: 43 g | Salt: 1.2 g

HIGH-KCAL | HIGH-CARB | HIGH-PROTEIN

1. Heat the olive oil in a large sauté pan. Add the mince and brown for 8–10 minutes.

2. While the mince is browning, place the lentils in a saucepan. Make up a quick chicken stock with the stock cube and boiling water. Transfer to the pan with the lentils and simmer for 15 minutes or until the lentils have absorbed the liquid.

3. Add the onions and garlic purée to the mince and cook for a further 5 minutes. Stir the passata and lentil mix into the mince. Season well and simmer for 10 minutes.

4. Serve with the pasta of your choice.

Stretch cottage pie

This is probably the tastiest and simplest cottage pie you will ever make. If you're totally wrecked from riding your bike real hard, use pre-prepared diced veg. Gravy granules as opposed to making a stock or any such nonsense make this dish the ultimate low-stress, full-flavour comfort food.

Serves 2

1 tablespoon olive oil

200 g (7 oz) mixed diced vegetables (carrot, parsnip, onion, butternut squash)

150 ml (⅔ cup) water

2 tablespoons gravy granules

100 g (3½ oz) frozen peas

300 g (11 oz) Stretch lentil and beef Bolognese (*see* p. 159)

sea salt and freshly ground black pepper

375 g (13 oz) mashed potato

Nutrition per serving:
Energy: 602 kcal
Total carbohydrate: 71 g (of which sugars: 16 g)
Fat: 20 g (of which saturates: 8.7 g)
Fibre: 11 g | Protein: 27 g | Salt: 3.6 g

HIGH-KCAL | HIGH-CARB | HIGH-PROTEIN

1. Heat the oil in a large heavy-based saucepan. Add the vegetables and cook over a medium heat for 5–6 minutes. Stir in the water, simmer and then stir in the gravy granules until you have a sticky vegetable mix.

2. Stir the peas and mince into the vegetables and simmer for 10–15 minutes. Adjust the seasoning.

3. Transfer to an ovenproof dish, allow to cool and then place in the fridge for 30 minutes to firm up – this makes it easier to top with mashed potato. It's easier to spread the mashed potato if you soften it by warming it through briefly in the oven or a microwave first.

4. Preheat the oven to 200°C/400°F/Gas 6. Place the dish in the centre of the oven and bake for 15–20 minutes. You can also brown the top under a hot grill if you are feeling 'cheffy'.

Stretch Moroccan mince

Finding a really good spice mix is key here. If you can take the time to source some good-quality za'atar spice or ras-el-hanout then the overall quality of the dish will be greatly improved as the flavours are so much better than generic supermarket dried spices.

Serves 2

1 teaspoon olive oil

1 pepper (any colour), deseeded and finely chopped

½ onion, peeled and finely chopped

1 tablespoon Moroccan seasoning

1 tin chickpeas (400 g/14 oz)

300 g (11 oz) Stretch lentil and beef Bolognese (*see* p. 159)

4 toasted pitta breads or cooked rice (allow 50 g/2 oz dry-weight per person) to serve

1. Warm the olive oil in a sauté pan. Add the pepper and onion. Cook over a medium heat for 2–3 minutes.

2. Sprinkle in the Moroccan seasoning, stir and cook for a further 2 minutes.

3. Stir in the chickpeas and simmer for 2 minutes before adding the Bolognese and heating through until piping hot.

4. Serve with toasted pittas or if you fancy more carbs, a side of cooked rice.

Nutrition per serving (with 2 pittas per person):
Energy: 762 kcal
Total carbohydrate: 114 g (of which sugars: 17 g)
Fat: 11 g (of which saturates: 2.3 g)
Fibre: 15 g | Protein: 43 g | Salt: 2.1 g

HIGH-KCAL | HIGH-CARB | HIGH-PROTEIN

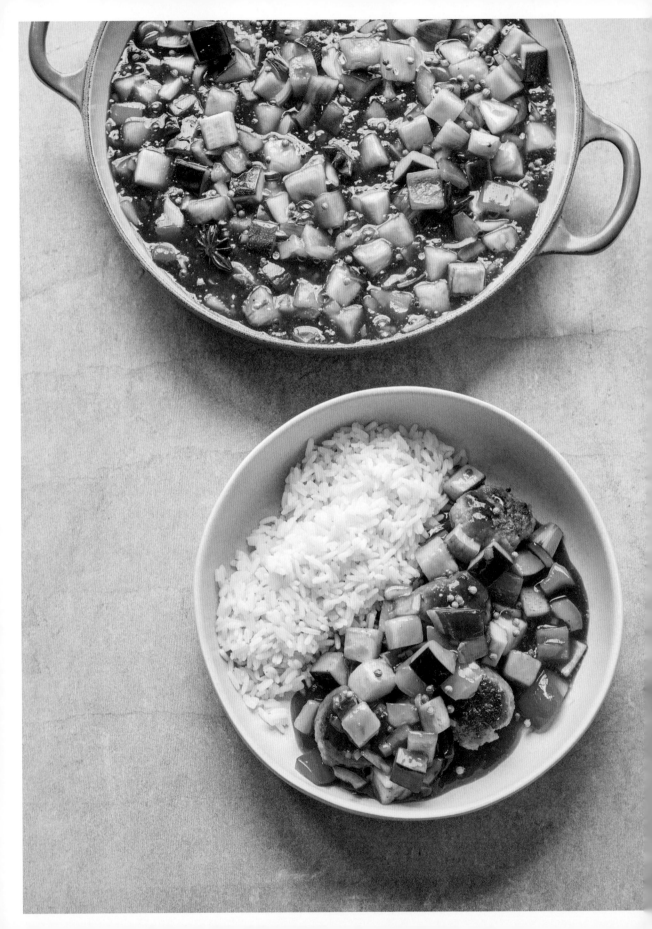

Pineapple and ginger sweet and sour

Full on flavour, perfect after a full-on bike day! This recipe packs a big carb punch so it's also great as a pre-loader the night before a monster ride. Pineapple and ginger sounds more like a dessert than a main course, but trust me on this one. The warmth of the ginger works so well with the sweetness of the pineapple juice. If you fancy spicing it up a little, you can always add a touch of fresh chilli. The dish also works brilliantly with turkey mince.

Serves 3… 2 portions for a main meal with 1 portion left for lunch the next day

500 g (1 lb 2 oz) pork mince

1 free-range egg

1 tablespoon flour

1 teaspoon lazy chilli

1 teaspoon ground ginger

pinch of sea salt and freshly ground black pepper

1 tablespoon olive oil

boiled rice to serve (Jasmine works particularly well here, allow 75 g (3 oz) dry-weight per person)

Sauce

2 tablespoons cornflour

4 tablespoons cold water

320 ml (1½ cups) pineapple juice

160 ml (⅔ cup) white wine vinegar

140 g (5 oz) honey

90 g (3½ oz) tomato ketchup

30 ml (1½ tablespoons) soy sauce

2 star anises

1 teaspoon coriander seeds

pinch of cinnamon

40 g (1½ oz) fresh grated ginger

Veggies

1 red, yellow and green pepper, deseeded and diced

1 large red onion, peeled and diced

1 medium courgette, trimmed, deseeded and diced

1 small aubergine, trimmed, deseeded and diced

200 g (7 oz) fresh pineapple, diced

1. First, make the roux. In a small bowl, mix together the cornflour and cold water with a fork to form a paste.

2. Combine all the remaining sauce ingredients in a saucepan and bring gently to the boil. Simmer for 2 minutes, stirring occasionally.

3. Whisk your roux again, then whisk gradually into the sauce mixture. Simmer gently for 3–4 minutes until it thickens, then stir in the diced vegetables and pineapple; set aside.

4. For the meatballs, mix all the ingredients with the exception of the oil together in a large bowl. Once well-combined, shape into 50 g (2 oz) balls with your palms.

5. To cook the meatballs, take a large sauté pan and add the oil. Heat it up and then, over a medium heat, fry the meatballs for 6–8 minutes, turning frequently until golden brown and cooked through.

6. Gently heat up the sweet and sour sauce, remove the star anises and serve the sauce with the meatballs on a bed of cooked rice.

Nutrition per serving:
Energy: 1038 kcal
Total carbohydrate: 147 g (of which sugars: 70 g)
Fat: 25 g (of which saturates: 7.6 g)
Fibre: 11 g | Protein: 48 g | Salt: 2.4 g

HIGH-KCAL | VERY-HIGH-CARB | HIGH-PROTEIN

Turkey 'Keith Reynolds'

Keith is the logistics manager for British Cycling. He's also an Olympian and former Commonwealth Games gold medallist and has some pedigree on the bike, it's safe to say! I once bodged this dish together on a camp and it was an instant hit – Keith asks for it every time.

It's nigh on impossible to make the small amount required here. The coriander pesto makes enough for 10 portions so divide it up and freeze any left over. Best frozen in individual portions for ease of use, and it keeps for 4–6 weeks. If you want to make it a real carb fest, serve with cooked rice (75 g/3 oz dry-weight per person).

Serves 2

500 g (1 lb 2 oz) turkey breast steaks

Coriander pesto

2 large bunches (200 g/7 oz) fresh coriander

75 g (3 oz) fresh ginger, peeled

2 garlic cloves, peeled

400 ml (1½ cups) olive oil

sea salt and freshly ground black pepper

Vegetable slaw

2 carrots, trimmed and peeled

1 courgette, trimmed

1 green pepper, deseeded

1 red onion, peeled

1 large pak choi, trimmed

small bunch of spring onions, trimmed and finely chopped, to finish

Dressing

2 tablespoons soy sauce,

2 tablespoons sesame oil

juice of 1 lime

1 tablespoon fresh ginger, grated

1. First, make your dressing for the slaw: in a small jug, mix the soy sauce, sesame oil, lime juice and grated ginger; stir well.

2. Into a large bowl, grate the carrots and courgette. Finely slice the pepper, onion and pak choi, add to the bowl and mix together.

3. Stir in the dressing, sprinkle over the spring onions and set aside.

4. For the coriander pesto, place the coriander, ginger, garlic, olive oil and seasoning in the bowl of a food processor and blend until smooth.

5. Now for the turkey steaks… Preheat your grill to a medium heat. Place the steaks on a non-stick baking tray and pour over a quarter of the coriander pesto. Leave to marinate for 10–15 minutes at room temperature before grilling for 3–4 minutes on each side.

6. Serve the turkey steaks on a bed of vegetable slaw. Drizzle over a little extra pesto to taste.

Nutrition per serving:
Energy: 998 kcal
Total carbohydrate: 23 g (of which sugars: 19 g)
Fat: 56 g (of which saturates: 8.5 g)
Fibre: 10 g | Protein: 96 g | Salt: 2.6 g

HIGH-KCAL | LOW-CARB | HIGH-PROTEIN

Thai-spiced coconut broth

Big flavour, big calories… perfect for after a big old day! This Thai-style dish is a favourite in our house and can be made up in advance. It also freezes well. You can replace the shrimps and salmon with 500 g (1 lb 2 oz) diced chicken. If you do that, increase the cooking time by 6 minutes. You can reduce the calories by using light coconut milk.

Serves 4

1 tablespoon olive oil

100 g (3½ oz) fresh ginger, finely chopped

1 small fresh chilli, deseeded

2 sticks of lemongrass, finely chopped

2 tablespoons Thai green curry paste

800 ml (3¼ cups) coconut milk

400 ml (1½ cups) chicken or fish stock

2 tablespoons Thai fish sauce and a little extra for seasoning

juice of 1 lime

400 g (14 oz) fresh salmon, cut into large dice

160 g (5½ oz) cooked shrimps

600 g (1¼ lb) mixed vegetables (pak choi, baby corn, mangetouts, baby spinach, courgettes, green beans)

1 bunch of fresh coriander, chopped

boiled rice to serve (allow 75 g (3 oz) dry-weight per person – Jasmine works particularly well with this recipe)

1. Heat the oil in a large non-stick saucepan, then add the ginger, chilli, lemongrass and curry paste. Cook over a low heat for 4–5 minutes.

2. Stir in the coconut milk and stock. Simmer for 15 minutes before seasoning with the fish sauce and lime juice.

3. Add the salmon, shrimps and vegetables and simmer for 3–4 minutes.

4. Adjust the seasoning again by adding a little more Thai fish sauce, if required, then sprinkle with coriander and serve with rice.

Nutrition per serving:
Energy: 1106 kcal
Total carbohydrate: 111 g (of which sugars: 40 g)
Fat: 56 g (of which saturates: 37 g)
Fibre: 6.5 g | Protein: 36 g | Salt: 5.5 g

VERY-HIGH-KCAL | HIGH-CARB | HIGH-PROTEIN

'St Clements' cod and pickled veg escabeche

Citrus and fish is a natural marriage. The pickled veg mixture is best made up in advance to allow the flavours to infuse – ideally, do this the day before and store it in the fridge. Escabeche means 'cooked' in vinegar and is a Mediterranean style of cooking. This light dish can be carbed up with the addition of some new potatoes and would work well with pretty much any fish and also grilled scallops.

Serves 2

2 x 150 g (5 oz) cod fillet

Citrus/oil/vegetable mix

1 large courgette, trimmed and grated

1 large carrot, trimmed, peeled and grated

1 large red onion, peeled and finely sliced

1 fennel bulb, trimmed and finely sliced

500 ml (2 cups) fresh orange juice

juice of 2 lemons and 2 limes

75 ml (4½ tablespoons) extra virgin olive oil

sea salt and freshly ground black pepper

1 bunch of basil, shredded

Marinade

1 teaspoon olive oil

1 teaspoon black onion seeds

2 teaspoons lemon juice

1 teaspoon lime juice

1. Place all the prepared vegetables in a large heatproof bowl.

2. Add the citrus juices to a medium saucepan. Reduce by half, then stir in the extra virgin olive oil and simmer for 2 minutes.

3. Pour the hot citrus oil mix on to the vegetables and stir well. Season and set aside to cool. Once cooled, stir in the basil and leave to infuse at room temperature for 30 minutes.

4. Strain off the citrus/vegetable liquor into a pan and over a low heat reduce slowly to form a dressing-like consistency. Set aside.

5. Mix together the olive oil, onion seeds, lemon and lime juices in a large mixing bowl. Add the cod and marinate for 15 minutes. Meanwhile, preheat a grill and get it nice and hot. Place the cod in an ovenproof dish with the citrus juice mixture, season well and grill for 6–7 minutes, basting with the juices.

6. Once the fish is cooked, serve with the pickled vegetables and some of the citrus dressing.

Nutrition per serving:
Energy: 653 kcal
Total carbohydrate: 36 g (of which sugars: 32 g)
Fat: 39 g (of which saturates: 5.7 g)
Fibre: 7.1 g | Protein: 32 g | Salt: 0.69 g

HIGH-KCAL | MEDIUM-CARB | HIGH-PROTEIN

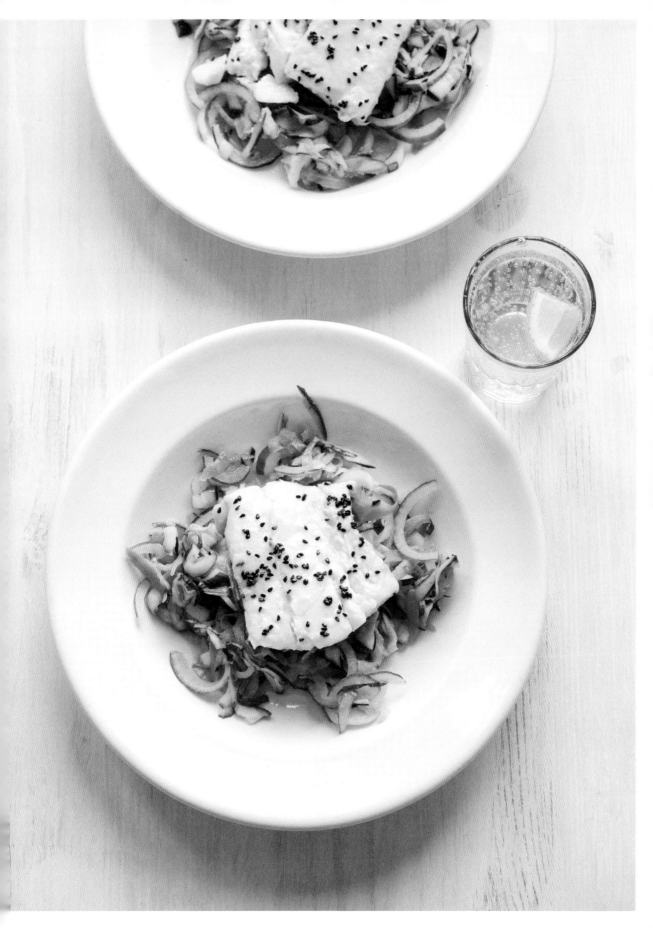

Smoked paprika, tomato and thyme meatballs

This meal can be low- to medium-carb depending on your ride intensity or duration. A good spicy meatball is hard to beat! Personally, I love the flavour profile of smoked paprika and, with a touch of BBQ spices, you have a winning combo. Turkey mince is a welcome change from traditional beef and is lower in fat so ideal when counting calories.

If you are serving the meatballs with pasta, you can do this in the time it takes to simmer the sauce and cook the meatballs (pasta usually takes 8–10 minutes but check the directions on the pack).

Serves 2 with a portion left for lunch

500 g (1 lb 2 oz) turkey breast mince

1 large onion, peeled and finely chopped

75 g (3 oz) fresh breadcrumbs

1 medium free-range egg

1 tablespoon plain flour

2 tablespoons smoked paprika

2 teaspoons BBQ spices

sea salt and freshly ground black pepper

1 tablespoon olive oil

Sauce

1 teaspoon smoked paprika

1 large red pepper, deseeded and sliced

1 large red onion, peeled and finely sliced

1 teaspoon chopped garlic

1 tin (400 g/14 oz) chopped tomatoes

1 bunch of fresh thyme (pick off the leaves)

spaghetti, if liked, to serve (allow 75 g/ 3 oz dry-weight per person)

1. Make the meatballs up by mixing all the ingredients together except for the oil and season well. Roll with your hands into 50–60 g (2–2½ oz) balls and set aside.

2. Preheat a large sauté pan and add the oil. Fry the meatballs over a medium heat for 3–4 minutes until golden brown. Leave the oil in the pan to make the sauce but transfer the meatballs to a baking tray.

3. Preheat the oven to 190°C/375°F/Gas 5… and wait! Don't put the meatballs in yet.

4. Now get your sauce on! Using the same pan as the one for the meatballs, add the paprika, peppers, onion and garlic. Mix together and cook, stirring, over a low heat for 5 minutes.

5. Add the chopped tomatoes, season and stir in the fresh thyme. Simmer for 10 minutes – enough time for you to cook the meatballs for 8 minutes in the centre of the oven. Serve with spaghetti, if liked.

Nutrition per serving (with pasta):
Energy: 764 kcal
Total carbohydrate: 95 g (of which sugars: 19 g)
Fat: 13 g (of which saturates: 2.9 g)
Fibre: 13 g | Protein: 59 g | Salt: 0.95 g

HIGH-KCAL | HIGH-CARB | HIGH-PROTEIN

Nutrition per serving (without pasta):
Energy: 503 kcal
Total carbohydrate: 44 g (of which sugars: 17 g)
Fat: 12 g (of which saturates: 2.7 g)
Fibre: 9.5 g | Protein: 50 g | Salt: 0.93 g

MEDIUM-KCAL | MEDIUM-CARB | HIGH-PROTEIN

Virgin Puttanesca

Whiter than white... This tasty yet simple pasta dish is a hit with the whole family. Serve with a green salad to add extra nutrients.

Serves 2

200 g (7 oz) gluten-free or regular spaghetti

1 lemon

200 ml (¾ cup) low-fat crème fraîche

200 g (7 oz) smoked salmon, chopped

2 tablespoons mini capers

small bunch of chopped dill

sea salt and freshly ground black pepper

Nutrition per serving:
Energy: 705 kcal
Total carbohydrate: 74 g (of which sugars: 5.9 g)
Fat: 27 g (of which saturates: 13 g)
Fibre: 4.3 g | Protein: 39 g | Salt: 3.7 g

HIGH-KCAL | HIGH-CARB | HIGH-PROTEIN

1. Cook the spaghetti according to the instructions on the pack.

2. Meanwhile, grate the zest of the lemon into a medium saucepan. Stir in the crème fraîche, smoked salmon pieces and the lemon juice.

3. Gently heat through the creamy sauce and at the last minute, stir in the mini capers and chopped dill.

4. Stir through the cooked pasta, adjust the seasoning and transfer to warmed plates.

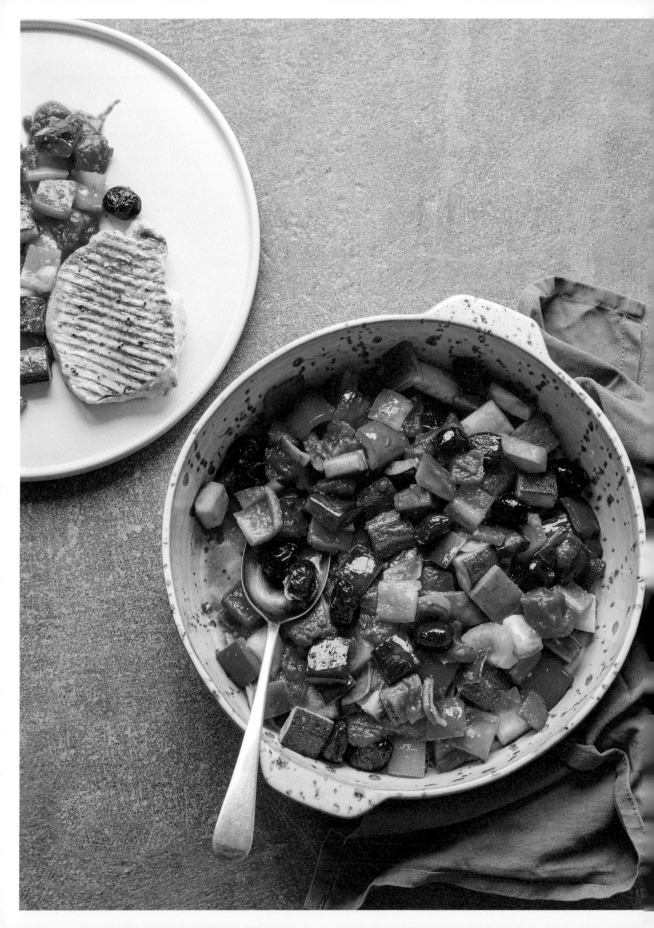

Ratatouille 'Murch-style' with lean pork chops

Ratatouille cooked properly is a fine thing. However, it's all too easy to throw a load of veg in a pan and end up with a mushy, over-cooked mess. My method works better as each of the veggies used is best cooked separately and then brought together at the last minute for a far nicer texture and fresher flavour.

Serves 4

2 courgettes

1 large red onion, peeled

1 red pepper

1 yellow pepper

1 green pepper

1 large aubergine

4 garlic cloves

2 tablespoons olive oil for the vegetables and 1 teaspoon olive oil for the meat

sea salt and freshly ground black pepper

1 tin (400 g/14 oz) chopped tomatoes

75 g (3 oz) good-quality pitted black olives

750 g (1½ lb) pork loin chops (allow 2 chops per person, about 150 g/5 oz each)

Nutrition per serving:
Energy: 710 kcal
Total carbohydrate: 13 g (of which sugars: 12 g)
Fat: 54 g (of which saturates: 17 g)
Fibre: 6.6 g | Protein: 39 g | Salt: 0.71 g

HIGH-KCAL | LOW-CARB | HIGH-PROTEIN

1. Spend some time dicing all the veggies evenly into medium chunks so they are roughly the same size. Keep separate, apart from the peppers, which can be mixed together. Remember to deseed too. Peel and finely slice the garlic.

2. Take 1 tablespoon of the olive oil and coat the aubergine in it, season well and set aside. Add a touch of the remaining oil to each of the veggies to coat. Cook each of the oil-coated vegetables and the garlic in a large saucepan and set aside (you can use the same pan, no need to wash it between veg). Cooking times as follows:

   • Courgettes over a medium heat for 2 minutes
   • Onions and garlic over a high heat for 3–4 minutes
   • Peppers over a medium heat for 5 minutes
   • Aubergine over a medium heat for 5–6 minutes

3. Once the veggies are all cooked, season well and return to the pan. Stir in the chopped tomatoes and olives. Simmer for no more than 5 minutes.

4. Meanwhile, preheat the grill to medium. Lightly brush the pork chops with olive oil. Season well and grill for 2–3 minutes on each side. Serve with the ratatouille.

Green sauce with tatties

Give this carb-based meal that can be prepared ahead a go. Salsa verde simply means 'green sauce'. Variations can be found pretty much anywhere from Mexico to mainland Europe. It's essentially a great way of using up an abundance of herbs when in season and the addition of capers/gherkins/vinegar/mustard lends a touch of welcome acidity.

The salsa can be served with lamb, fish or even just tossed through a salad of mixed vegetables. It is pretty tricky to make up a small amount so make a batch (the recipe makes 8–10 portions) and keep in the fridge for up to 2 weeks. Or take some to your neighbours – everyone loves a food gift!

Serves 2

500 g (1 lb 2 oz) new potatoes,
cut in half

2 hot smoked salmon fillets (180 g/6 oz
per person)

Salsa (1 tablespoon per person)

1 garlic clove

1 bunch each parsley, mint and basil

1 tablespoon capers

1 tablespoon pickled gherkins

4 anchovies

150 ml (⅔ cup) extra virgin olive oil

2 teaspoons white wine vinegar

1 tablespoon Dijon mustard

Nutrition per serving:
Energy: 645 kcal
Total carbohydrate: 39 g (of which sugars: 5.6 g)
Fat: 30 g (of which saturates: 5.6 g)
Fibre: 4.8 g | Protein: 51 g | Salt: 4.2 g

HIGH-KCAL | MEDIUM-CARB | HIGH-PROTEIN

1. Simmer the potatoes in boiling salted water until softened, about 10–15 minutes. Cover to keep warm and set aside.

2. To make the salsa, blend all the ingredients in the bowl of a food processor to make a smooth paste.

3. Stir 2–3 tablespoons salsa into the potatoes, ideally when they are still warm from cooking.

4. Serve the potatoes with the hot smoked salmon.

Hardcore pre-bed chocolate bircher muesli

Excellent after a hard ride to aid recovery, this take on a classic bircher muesli is also good when you have a late-night training session and can't face a meal, or if you raced in the evening.

Chocolate and vanilla in any format work so well. This snack-type meal is very much one to keep in the bank for those tougher rides or when you have multiple long/hard back-to-back days planned and having a pre-bed meal makes complete sense when you are ruined. The recipe contains a whole load of calories so make sure you use it carefully!

Makes 1 portion

90 g (3½ oz) chocolate milk

75 g (3 oz) low-fat yoghurt

50 g (2 oz) gluten-free oats

30 g (1¼ oz) vanilla whey protein

1 teaspoon chia

1 tablespoon puffed quinoa

1 tablespoon mixed seeds

Nutrition per serving:
Energy: 557 kcal
Total carbohydrate: 59 g (of which sugars: 17 g)
Fat: 14 g (of which saturates: 3.1 g)
Fibre: 7.5 g | Protein: 46 g | Salt: 0.39 g

HIGH-KCAL | HIGH-CARB | HIGH-PROTEIN

1. Mix all ingredients together in a bowl, cover and place in the fridge for 30 minutes. Stir the mix just before serving and enjoy!

Chickpea mocha brownies

These brownies are ideal for snacking because, being quite rich, you don't need to eat too big a portion – perfect for on the bike or as a pre-ride snack. Or try one of these bad boys chopped up and mixed with a large spoonful of Greek yoghurt for dessert. It's snacking that's good for vegan types, too, as no coconuts were harmed in the development of this recipe.

Makes 24 x 35 g (1½ oz) bars (snack-size)

400 g (14 oz) chickpeas, strained

250 g (9 oz) Medjool dates

120 g (4 oz) crunchy nut butter

90 g (3½ oz) coconut oil, melted

1 teaspoon vanilla extract

pinch of sea salt

50 g (2 oz) cocoa powder

2 teaspoons good-quality instant coffee (optional)

30 g (1¼ oz) cocoa nibs

60 g (2½ oz) walnuts

Nutrition per serving:
Energy: 144 kcal
Total carbohydrate: 10 g (of which sugars: 7.2 g)
Fat: 9.5 g (of which saturates: 4.6 g)
Fibre: 2.1 g | Protein: 3.4 g | Salt: 0.05 g

MEDIUM-KCAL | MEDIUM-CARB | LOW-PROTEIN

1. Fit a food processor with the paddle attachment and into the bowl add the chickpeas, dates, nut butter, coconut oil, vanilla extract and salt. Beat until fairly smooth.

2. Gradually add the cocoa powder, coffee (if using) and the cocoa nibs until the mixture forms a paste.

3. Finally, add the walnuts and whizz for 20 seconds max to ensure the texture of the nuts is retained.

4. Transfer the mixture to a 22 x 22 cm (9 x 9 in) tin and smooth with a palette knife. Place in the fridge to set for 1 hour, then slice into bars. Store in the fridge for up to 2 weeks, although it's highly unlikely they will last that long!

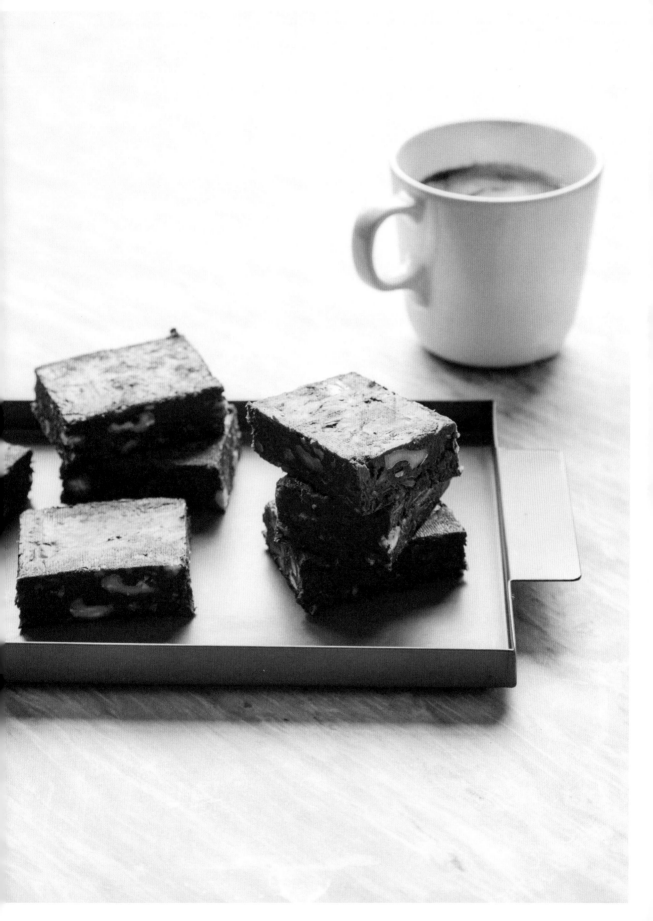

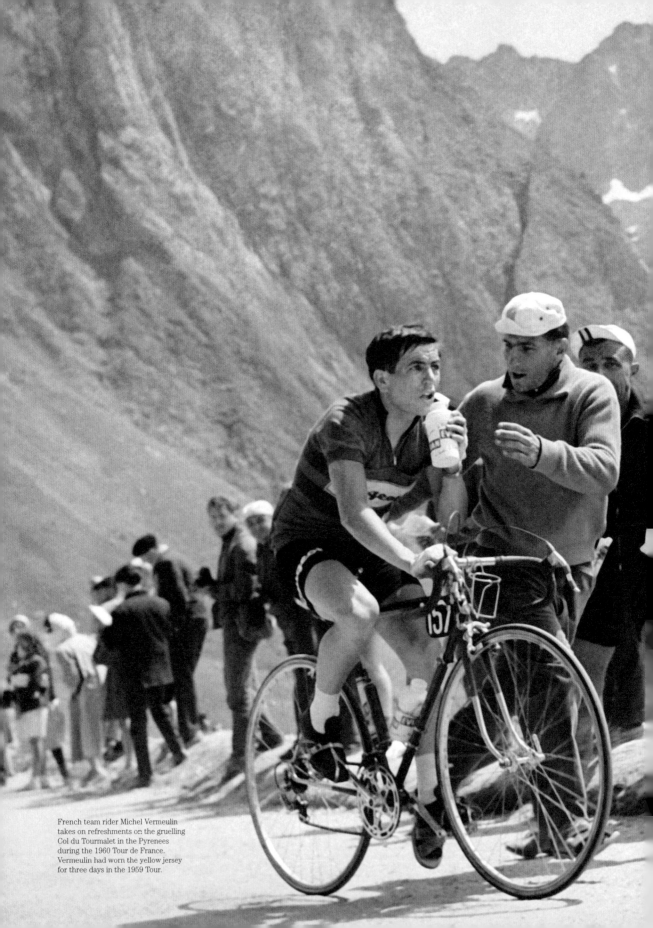

French team rider Michel Vermeulin
takes on refreshments on the gruelling
Col du Tourmalet in the Pyrenees
during the 1960 Tour de France.
Vermeulin had worn the yellow jersey
for three days in the 1959 Tour.

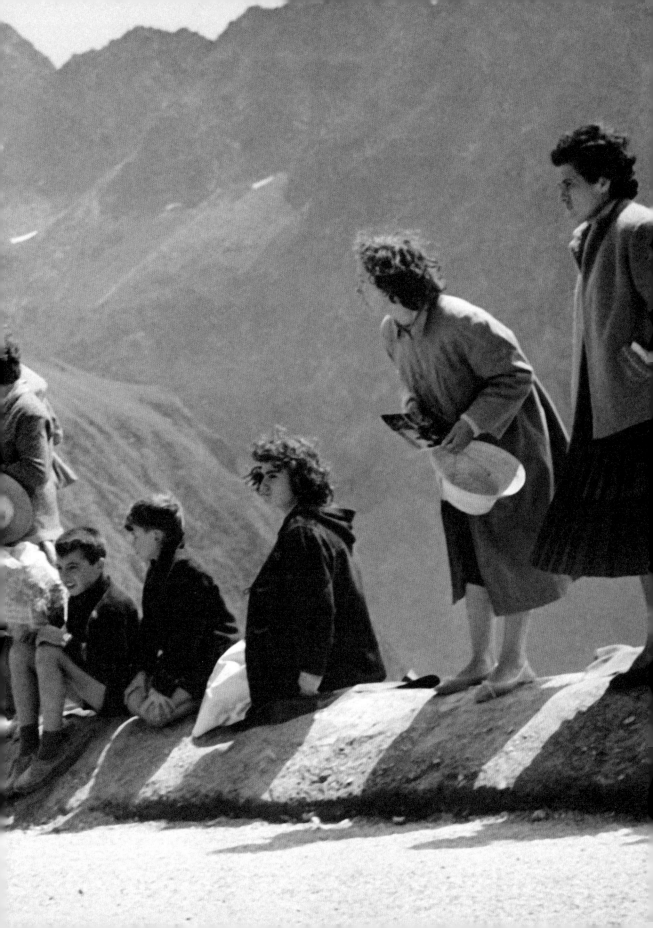

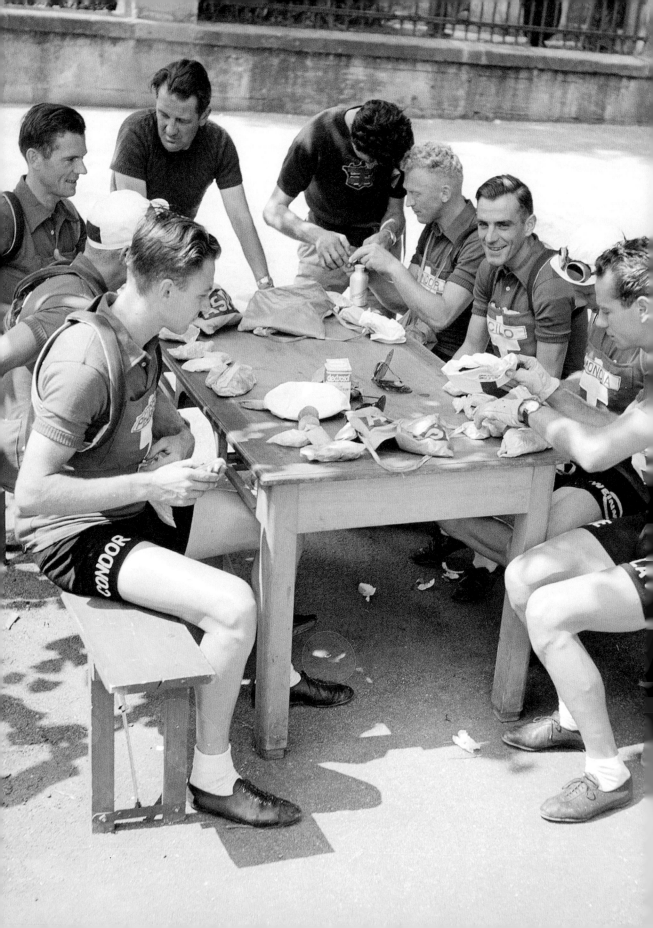

Meal Planner

Following a nutritional plan is every bit as important as sticking to a training schedule. Planning your meals will enable you to make sure your fuelling matches the intensity of your training and that you have the right levels of nutrients your body needs. In this chapter I have outlined some example meal planning for easy, medium and hard training days using recipes from this book. I have suggested a breakfast, lunch and evening meal, and included a snack option, which can be eaten to fill the gap mid-morning or mid-afternoon.

The Swiss team tuck in before the start of the 1951 Tour de France in Metz. Hugo Koblet (front right) would go on to win the race.

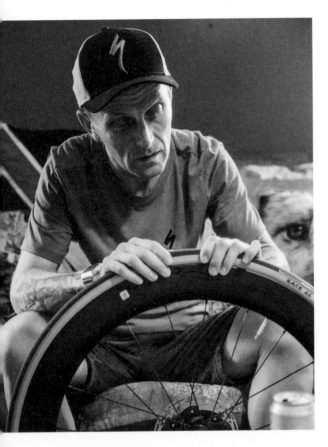

You can't always put your feet up on rest days as there are often chores to do – including bike maintenance. However, you can still make sure you eat well and prepare for harder days.

This is not a plan set in stone. We all have different basal metabolic rates (the amount of energy you need to take in simply to stay alive) and on top of your training load for the day you will also experience differing levels of daily stressors, which have a huge impact on your food requirements. If you are in a manual job, for example, you will have far greater energy requirements than your more sedentary counterparts. How much sleep you achieved the night before also has an impact on appetite. If you feel you need larger or smaller portions than those specified, then you're probably right!

Rest day

Ideally, rest days are all about chilling out and repairing those tired muscles ready for another epic ride or adventure in the coming days. In reality this is not often the case. Rest days are often taken up with fulfilling family obligations, catching up on work, having a social life and all the other things that make us a balanced human being. My rest day menu here is high on taste, lighter on calories, but still packs in seven servings of fruit or veg and is loaded with appetite-satisfying protein sources. We start the day with a high-protein low-carb number using duck eggs and ricotta, along with vitamin-rich spinach and mushrooms. This will set you up well and help keep you going until lunch when you will be tucking into my Easy tomato and basil soup, which can be made up in advance and batch-cooked – perfectly portable to take into the office if you are working that day. If you're feeling extra-hungry, add some good-quality sourdough bread for a carb boost. Fill the mid-afternoon lull with a protein pot: here, I have suggested the Beetroot, feta and chickpea hummus pot, but you can choose from any of the protein pots listed in this book (*see* pp. 90-94). Finish the day strong with a refreshing, crisp Watermelon, feta and Serrano ham salad, which is sweet and salty and gives a really interesting textural eating experience. Beats the cottage cheese and rice cake diet, hey?

Easy day

Your energy requirements on an easy day will only be marginally higher than a rest day, but you may have a bit more of an appetite due to the hunger-boosting impact of training. The Matcha oat breakfast smoothie is more like a meal in a glass and far more satisfying than any pre-packaged fruit smoothie, which are often purely simple carb-based. Matcha is a type of Japanese green tea and boasts a host of benefits, including improving mental clarity, which makes it a perfect way to kick off your day. For lunch, I have suggested Sweet potato tortilla, Vittoria-style, which needs just four ingredients, can be made up in advance and, it goes without saying, is super tasty! The perfect combo of slow-release carbs and protein to fuel your easy spin. In the evening you will be tucking into Baked ginger and sesame sea bream 'en papillote' – a fancy way of saying baked fish in paper. Not quite fish and chips, but I think you'll agree it's worth the effort. For those in-between energy slumps or as a snack before or after your ride, make up a batch of Cherry coconut granola bars. Serve simply on its own or with a good dollop of Greek yoghurt and berries – happy snacking!

Medium day

Medium training days are always a tricky balance between eating enough to support your training, and overestimating your energy burn and emptying the contents of the fridge when you get in from your ride. The key to getting this right is forward planning. Eating well throughout the day will lessen the urge cram in calories post-ride as you will not feel physically or psychologically depleted. I have kept the food interesting in terms of flavours and textures to satisfy taste buds as well as muscles!

Start the day right with Cheeky cherry breakfast muffins. These are also ideal to eat while on your ride if you are the type of person who likes to get up and go in the early morning. This recipe is great to get little people involved with the household cooking and far superior in terms of taste and nutritional value than any shop-bought, processed equivalent. Lunching on a banging broth of chicken, mushroom and ginger will give you loads of flavour without upsetting the calorie balance for the day. Finish the day with Kofta-style turkey and ghetto slaw, which combines lean, sleep-inducing protein with a nitrate-boosting beetroot mixed with a host of raw veg – think very holistic kebab shop! My Chickpea mocha brownies will plug the gaps and as they use chickpeas, which are high in protein, as a base and have a rich chocolate flavour, you don't need to eat too big a portion, which helps you stick to your optimal energy target.

Hard day

When it comes to hard training days or races, what you eat the day before the event is as important as on the day itself. Head into a big day depleted and you are setting yourself up for failure at worst, or a longer day than anticipated in the saddle at best. Under fuel and you will leave yourself more susceptible to any bug making the rounds. Hard training days need fuel! This is the time to park any weight-loss ambitions on the bench and shift your focus to performance. You won't be able to complete really challenging training or racing on a deficit, so don't attempt to do so or you will sell yourself short. Keep in mind why you are training – to be the fastest cyclist you can be – weight loss can wait until tomorrow.

The day before a hard ride, focus on carbohydrate- and high-calorie dense foods. Pumpkin-spiced bircher muesli is a delicious take on classic bircher and feels like a real treat. Posh poached eggs with wild mushrooms and baby spinach served on good-quality sourdough is a simple, yet satisfying lunch with a perfect balance of carbs and protein. In the evening, top up the glycogen tanks with our soon-to-be cult classic, Pasta 'Barlow', inspired by international marathon runner Tracy Barlow – if anyone knows the importance of fuelling the machine, it's an elite marathoner. Using four simple ingredients, you can replicate this dish anywhere. High-carb, low-fibre and high in taste, it's perfect for the night before a big challenge when your tummy may be doing backflips with nerves or adrenalin. And look to 'Wonder Woman' bars for snacking options – these are to enjoyed by everyone, regardless of gender!

For the hard day itself, I recommend Raspberry-banana ripple-baked oats or any of the baked oats variations, if practical (*see* p. 153). However, if you have a really early-morning event, go with bircher again from the previous day. Once you go 'baked', you will never go back – you will never look at a pan of boiled porridge the same way again. Even being a hardened Scot, I rarely cook my porridge traditionally anymore. Nutty carrot slaw with edamame beans for lunch is a sweet and salty combo, which is equally good before or after your ride. You can add a lean protein – for example, grilled chicken – and serve with white rice for easy-to-digest carbs. Post-ride is time for a serious refuel and treat for a job well done. Granny-style Tikka 'tattie scones' with coconut lentil dahl is a not-so-dirty curry but still feels like a real indulgence with its feel-good flavours – a more cyclist-friendly alternative to your standard takeaway. For the race itself, Cheryl's coconut oat balls are ideal for topping up the tanks before, during or after the ride. They are a neutral flavour and jersey-pocket friendly, making them the perfect ride fuel.

And if you are still hungry after all that, Pre-bed chia puddings with sour cherry and almond are a cyclist super-dessert. Taking inspiration from the traditional cherry bakewell, this pre-bed snack gives tired muscles a much-needed protein hit as well as helping an exhausted brain to wind down and get some vitamin Z, with the aid of the sleep-inducing properties of sour cherries.

I think you'll agree this menu is a real incentive to plan those hard rides in!

Sample Meal Planner

In creating recipes for this book, I tested them rigorously on the harshest food critics – teenagers and athletes. Myself, my partner, who is also a cyclist, and my teenage girls all sit down to eat these meals together and we can tweak them to meet individual requirements. Sometimes we have different macronutrient requirements depending on the duration and intensity of our training so we can adjust the protein/carb ratios accordingly. On the following pages are a couple of typical food days in the Performance Chef household. With the dual focus of meeting your needs as a cyclist and providing interesting flavours and textures, everyone is a winner!

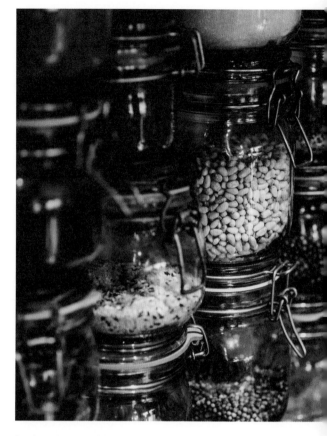

Boredom is the enemy of the healthy eater. Having a variety of ingredients on hand is essential to ensuring your diet remains interesting, tasty and nutritional.

Cheryl's coconut oat balls are ideal for topping up the tanks before, during or after the ride. They are a neutral flavour and jersey-pocket friendly, making them the perfect ride fuel.

Sample 1

	Rest Day	Easy Training Day	Medium Training Day	Pre-hard Day	Hard Ride or Race
Breakfast	Baked duck eggs with spinach, ricotta and wild mushrooms (*see* p. 60)	Matcha oat breakfast smoothie (*see* p. 76)	Cheeky cherry breakfast muffins (*see* p. 128)	Pumpkin-spiced bircher muesli (*see* p. 106)	Raspberry-banana ripple-baked oats (*see* p. 152)
Lunch	Easy tomato and basil soup (*see* p. 53)	Sweet potato tortilla, Vittoria-style (*see* p. 82)	Banging broth of chicken, mushroom and ginger (*see* p. 135)	Posh poached eggs with wild mushrooms and baby spinach (*see* p. 142)	Nutty carrot slaw with edamame beans (*see* p. 110)
Dinner	Watermelon, feta and Serrano ham salad (*see* p. 64)	Baked ginger and sesame sea bream 'en papillote' (*see* p. 88)	Kofta-style turkey and ghetto slaw (*see* p. 132)	Pasta 'Barlow' (*see* p. 113)	Tikka 'tattie scones' with coconut lentil dahl (*see* p. 156)
Snacking	Beetroot, feta and chickpea hummus protein pot (*see* p. 92)	Cherry coconut granola bars (*see* p. 130)	Chickpea mocha brownies (*see* p. 174)	'Wonder Woman' bars (*see* p. 143)	Cheryl's coconut oat balls (*see* p. 108)
Pre-bed					Pre-bed chia puddings with sour cherry and almond (*see* p. 116)

Sample 2

	Rest Day	Easy Training Day	Medium Training Day	Pre-hard Day	Hard Ride or Race
Breakfast	Poached red fruit with basil and pink peppercorns (*see* p. 95) served with low-fat Greek yoghurt	DIY muesli (*see* p. 78) served with oat milk	Ginger-spiced granola with cinnamon and black pepper (*see* p. 52) served with Greek yoghurt	Cherry 'baked well' oats (*see* p. 154)	Apple strudel flavour baked oats (*see* p. 155)
Lunch	Thai-style beef and raw vegetable salad (*see* p. 58)	Roasted butternut squash and beetroot salad (*see* p. 77)	Two-for-one 'Murch magic' mushroom soup (*see* p. 81) served with sourdough	French toast sandwich with smoked ham and grainy mustard (*see* p. 29)	Bonzer breakfast burrito (*see* p. 131)
Dinner	Baked cod with tomato ketchup and tarragon relish (*see* p. 59)	Chillin' (*see* p. 80) served with baked sweet potato	Risotto-ish with red lentils (*see* p. 112)	Two-for-one 'Murch magic' mushroom soup and pasta bake (*see* p. 81)	Za'atar roasted leg of lamb with pomegranate seeds, chickpeas and mint (*see* p. 30)
Snacking	Avocado, prawn and lemon protein pot (*see* p. 94)	Carrot and edamame protein pot (*see* p. 90)	Sweet potato tortilla, Vittoria-style (*see* p. 82)	Coconut, lemon curd and gingerbread chia puddings (*see* p. 42)	Cheeky cherry breakfast muffins (*see* p. 128)
Pre-bed					Hardcore pre-bed chocolate bircher muesli (*see* p. 173)

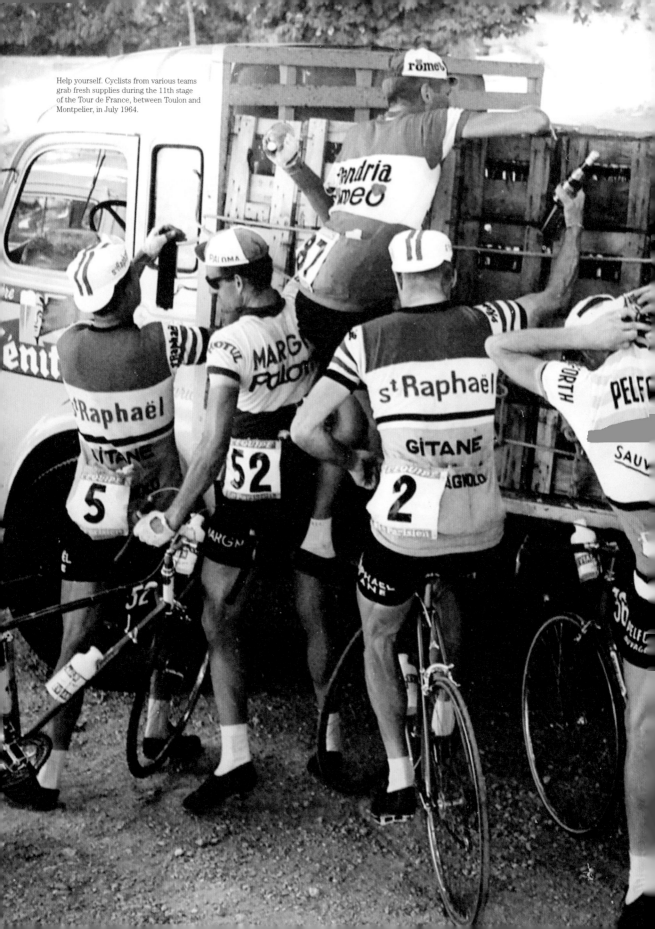

Help yourself. Cyclists from various teams grab fresh supplies during the 11th stage of the Tour de France, between Toulon and Montpelier, in July 1964.

Acknowledgements

First, a huge thank you to everyone who has bought and used my first book, *The Cycling Chef: Recipes for Performance and Pleasure*, as it was intended. Without that, this 'difficult second album' would have been a non-starter. The feedback and interaction via social media exceeded all my expectations by some way, so keep that shit up! Safe to say, this has been a tough book to write – new recipe development and re-inventing the metaphorical wheel in some respects has been a fair old challenge. Hence why I needed a pro-elite team of eager, hungry and willing recipe testers. A selfless (or should that be selfish?) act.

Chief testers, a big shout out: Elinor Barker, Alec Briggs, Anel Meyer, Ruth Astle, Hayley Simmonds, Kim Morrison, Ryan Owens, Chanel Harris, El Dickinson, Isabella Bertold, Jack Carlin, Oliver Bridgewood, Richard Cook, Katy Marchant, Ken Buckley, Alice Barnes, Alistair Donohue, Mummy Archibald, Mark Stewart, and I even got Ed Clancy cooking! Continual testing, feedback and tweaking – let's call it 'marginal grains' – was key to making sure it was right. Plan, practise, execute. Much like cycling, really.

A big high five to the good people at Specialized HQ, Drag2Zero and Endura for continued support with bikes and kit to keep an old man looking good on the bike – all show and minimal go! The very best kit means that cycling is just that bit more pleasurable.

Nerdy nutrition stuff is not my thing, so cheers to Ted Munson for saintly checking my ambiguous nutritional knowledge.

The home kitchen is where the magic happens. Vickster and the girls are normally at the front line of the mess and creative process involved in being a 'sometimes genius-mostly lunatic' cooking person. Thank you for the clean plates and constructive criticism.

The team at Bloomsbury have been absolute troopers in bringing all my incoherent ramblings together, so thank you to Matt Lowing and his team of worker bees, especially Queen Bee Holly Jarrald, who made sure we got it all across the line in time... just. A lot of patience and an awesome eye for food pics, as ever, from Clare Winfield, who's also an avid food taster. Plus cracking bike and home images by Dan Gould. Thanks also to Adrian Besley and Adam Ackworth.

About the Author

Alan Murchison is very much an 'unprofessional' cyclist and not even the best cyclist in his own house. A Michelin-starred chef with over 25 years' experience working in starred restaurants (he held a Michelin star for over a decade and had 4 AA Rosettes while executive chef at L'Ortolan restaurant in Berkshire), he is now retired from the world of fancy pants cooking. He is also a national level master's cyclist (has ridden 18 minutes for 10 miles!), ex-international endurance runner and multiple World and European age-group duathlon champion.

Alan provides bespoke nutritional support and cooking advice for athletes across several sports, although predominantly for cyclists. He is a consultant with British Cycling and works with athletes across a range of abilities, from first-timers looking to just complete an event to World Tour riders and current Olympic/World Champions.

@performance.chef

Index

References

1. https://www.nhs.uk/live-well/healthy-weight/bmi-calculator/
2. https://www.bmi-calculator.net/body-fat-calculator/
3. http://www.loughborough-sports-science.com/body-composition-test.html
4. https://www.bmj.com/rapid-response/2011/11/02/negative-energy-balance-needed-fat-loss
5. 'Study on food intake and energy expenditure during extreme sustained exercise: the Tour de France', https://pubmed.ncbi.nlm.nih.gov/2744926/
6. https://pubmed.ncbi.nlm.nih.gov/22150425/ and https://www.ncbi.nlm.nih.gov/pmc/articles/PMC4913918/
7. https://www.ncbi.nlm.nih.gov/pmc/articles/PMC3562955/
8. https://neurosciencenews.com/eating-pleasure-neuroscience-7345/
9. https://www.mountelizabeth.com.sg/healthplus/article/fat-burning-zone-heart-rate-to-lose-fat
10. https://bjsm.bmj.com/content/bjsports/53/10/655.full.pdf
11. https://www.britishcycling.org.uk/knowledge/nutrition/eating-on-bike/article/izn20150818-All-Cycling-Fasted-Morning-Rides-0
12. https://www.healthline.com/health/diet-and-weight-loss/how-often-should-i-weigh-myself and https://www.nhs.uk/news/obesity/weighing-yourself-every-day-may-help-with-weight-loss/
13. https://www.webmd.com/sleep-disorders/features/lack-of-sleep-weight-gain

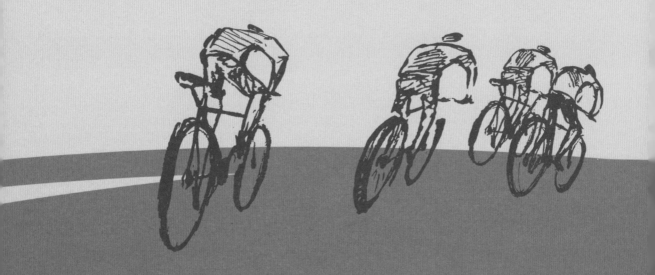